FOOD AND BEVERAGE CONSUMPTION AND HEALTH

PISUM SATIVUM

CULTIVATION, FUNCTIONAL PROPERTIES AND HEALTH BENEFITS

FOOD AND BEVERAGE CONSUMPTION AND HEALTH

Additional books in this series can be found on Nova's website under the Series tab.

Additional e-books in this series can be found on Nova's website under the e-book tab.

FOOD AND BEVERAGE CONSUMPTION AND HEALTH

PISUM SATIVUM

CULTIVATION, FUNCTIONAL PROPERTIES AND HEALTH BENEFITS

SHANNELL BECKET
EDITOR

NOVINKA
New York

Additional color graphics may be available in the e-book version of this book.

Library of Congress Cataloging-in-Publication Data

ISBN: 978-1-63463-230-0
Library of Congress Control Number: 2014952257

Published by Nova Science Publishers, Inc. † New York

CONTENTS

PREFACE

The pea *Pisum sativum* are rich in proteins and dietary fiber and contribute considerably to the total dietary protein requirements. Peas are abundant in complex carbohydrates giving rise to food with a low glycemic index. Peas are hypolipidemic. Fiber in peas contains more amylose than amylopectin and is antihyperglycemic. Peas can be used in processed foods such as bakery products, bread, snack foods, soups, and tortillas. Because of their nutritious value, it has been suggested that peas be included in snack foods, baby food, and sports food. This book discusses the cultivation of *Pisum sativum* as well as it's functional properties and health benefits.

Chapter 1 – Iron (Fe) participates in many essential plant functions, such as photosynthesis, respiration and nitrogen metabolism, including nodulation of legume plants. It is abundant in most soils but its availability is low, especially in calcareous soils (more than 30% of arable soils), where its solubility is very low and is frequent the incidence of Fe chlorosis. In these soils, one of the more important factors causing Fe chlorosis is bicarbonate while hypoxia, due to flooding or other causes, can aggravate its negative effects. According to the World Health Organization, the most common nutritional disorder in humans is Fe deficiency, with over 30% of the world's population affected. To solve both problems, two of the main objectives of plant Fe researchers are to obtain genotypes more efficient in Fe uptake (more tolerant to calcareous soils) and to get edible seeds with higher Fe content for human nutrition. For these goals, it is necessary to know better the mechanisms implicated in Fe uptake and their regulation. To acquire Fe from soils, plants have developed different strategies. Today, two main strategies are considered: the Strategy I, present in non graminaceous plants (dicots, non grasses monocots,…) and the Strategy II, present in graminaceous plants.

When plants suffer from Fe deficiency they switch on several morphological and physiological changes in their roots, known as Fe deficiency stress responses (hereafter named Fe responses), aimed to facilitate Fe acquisition and mobilization. These responses are switched off once plants acquire enough Fe, to avoid Fe intoxication and energy lost. Since pea is a dicot plant species, this review is devoted to describe the characteristics of Fe acquisition and Fe responses in Strategy I plants, pointing out the role of some pea mutants (*brz* and *dgl*) in the studies about this Strategy.

Chapter 2 – The pea *Pisum sativum* produces a diversity of enzymes and proteins. They include alpha-galactosidases, beta-galactosidase, insoluble acid invertase, germin-like protein with superoxide dismutase activity, glutathione reductase, aminoaldehyde dehydrogenase, NADP+-linked isocitrate dehydrogenase, p-aminobenzoylglutamate hydrolase, phospholipase C delta isoforms, cytoplasmic fructose-1,6-bisphosphatase, raffinose synthase, beta-ketoacyl-acyl carrier protein synthase III, caspases, DNA helicase 47, DNA helicase 45, chromatin-associated histone binding protein, beta-1,3-glucanase, symbiosis-related chitinases, Bowman-Birk protease inhibitors, angiotensin converting enzyme inhibitory peptide, antifungal proteins, C-6 oxidases, short-chain alcohol dehydrogenase-like protein, fatty acid alpha-dioxygenase, gibberellin dioxygenases, carbonic anhydrase, photosystem II proteins with carbonic anhydrase activity, C1 subgroup mitogen-activated protein kinase, Ca2+/calmodulin-dependent protein kinase, enzyme catalyzing conjugation of indole-3-acetic acid to aspartate, pea albumin 1F (PA1F), pea albumin 1, subunit b, vicilin, lectins, mitochondrial type II peroxiredoxin, channel-forming protein in chloroplasts, outer envelope membrane protein 16 of pea chloroplasts, cell wall fibronectin-like adhesion protein, arabinogalactanprotein-extensin glycoproteins, ferritin, and dehydrin.

Chapter 3 – Evidence has been presented that pea consumption may facilitate prevention of neural tube defects, increase of satiety and reduction of obesity, inhibition of atherosclerosis, prevention of cardiometabolic risk, reduction of head and neck cancer risk, lung cancer risk, colon cancer risk, reduction of fasting serum concentrations of adhesion molecules and inflammatory biomarkers. Pea has anti-oxidant, anti-inflammatory, immunomodulating, and angiotensin converting enzyme inhibitory activities. Trace elements such as selenium are rich in Canadian field peas, Peas may synergize with whole grains in health promoting effects.

Chapter 4 – A reactive oxygen species (ROS)-resistant *Pisum sativum* cv. 'Alaska' mutant, *R3-1,* has been reported as a double mutant of transit peptide-NDPK2 Ile12Leu and Lys205Glu and pre-sequence-NDPK3 Pro45Ser [Haque et al. (2010) *Planta* 232:367-382]. The yield of young pods was 2.1-fold higher in *R3-1* than that in the wild-type in the field of Kanagawa Agricultural Technology Center. The yield of plant weights in *R3-1* was 2.0-fold higher than those of the wild-type. The *R3-1* showed phenotypes of seedlings standing in the upward direction and the first leaf opening was very fast. In the case of wild-type the seedlings showed clear bending by fook formation. The *R3-1* mutant also showed slow growth in the upward direction, showing low response to negative gravitropism. The *R3-1* mutant showed a high temperature-resistant phenotype compared to that of wild-type, when the seedlings were grown at 35°C under illumination. The phosphorylation of soluble fractions in the wild type and the *R3-1* of leaves of field grown plants showed an increase in the high-molecular weight histidine kinases with molecular masses of 40, 48, 63 and 70 kDa in the mutant, and in the case of membrane fractions 63 and 72 kDa. The increase in the phosphorylation of these high-molecular weight histidine kinases may be the result of the photoresponses partly via the phytochrome, because the phytochrome mediated increase in the phosphorylation of NDPK2 was established. The molecular mechanisms including singlet oxygen and the resulting calcium release to cytosol from vacuole, microsome and plasma membranes were discussed.

Chapter 5 – To date, there is limited study on structural profiles on a molecular level mainly related to lipid biopolymers in different type of peas. This research aims to determine molecular structural features of lipid that mainly related to functional groups in the recently developed Green-type and Yellow-type CDC pea varieties: CDC Strike (Green-Type) vs. CDC Meadow (Yellow-Type) and relatively quantify the antisymmetric CH3 ("CH_3as") and CH2 ("CH_2as") (ca. 2960 and 2923 cm (-1), respectively), symmetric CH3 ("CH_3s") and CH2 ("CH_2s") (ca. 2873 and 2954 cm (-1), respectively) functional groups and carbonyl C=O ester (ca. 1745 cm (-1) spectral intensities as well as their ratios of antisymmetric CH(3) to antisymmetric CH(2) (Ratio of CH_3as to CH_2as), ratios of symmetric CH(3) to symmetric CH(2) (Ratio of CH_3s to CH_2s), and ratios of carbonyl C=O ester peak area to total CH peak area (Ratio of C=O ester to CH). Together with the multivariate molecular spectral analyses, the study focused on detecting spectral feature of molecular structure functional groups that are related to lipid biopolymer in different types of peas.

Chapter 6 – This review summarizes studies carried out on pea aphids, *Acyrtosiphon pisum* (Harris) (Aphididae: Homoptera) damaging food legumes in northwestern Ethiopia (much of the high plateau of the country is found here, over 2000 m above sea level) from 1998 to 2013. The review summarizes of various papers on pea aphids published in the area of wild legumes, aphid reproduction and survival, population dynamics, suitable weather conditions, host preference and evaluation of eco-friendly botanical products against aphids. During the initial studies, the author tried to identify how aphids over winter the rather long (9-month) dry season. It was found that wild leguminous plants such as clover, *Trifolium ruepellainum* and vetch, *Vicia* spp and the cultivated ones such as the perennial legumes (pigeon pea, *Cajanus cajan*) served as wild hosts. These are believed to sustain aphid survival during the dry season. In the greenhouse study, it was determined that the more the aphid density the lower the rate of reproduction and the longevity of aphids. Aphid population dynamics studies also showed that aphids prefer cool and dry climate, nevertheless warm episodes are necessary for reproduction. Lower altitudes are therefore found good hot-spots for the aphids. The author's research station (Adet Research Center, Amhara, Ethiopia) is located at 2240 m a.s.l. where the aphids are less important while 45 km north the altitude descends 400 m lower than our station, gets warmer and grass pea production has almost stopped there because of these aphids. Aphid numbers steadily increased from seedling stage to pod setting, and then drastically fell at maturity. Lentils and grass peas were more suitable hosts than faba bean and field pea. In Ethiopia, pea aphids were first reported in cool and dry regions of the extreme north, which later extended their range to even lower altitudes and warmer areas. Management studies carried out include botanicals, detergents, kerosene and some of the more conventional and aphid-specific pesticides. Promising botanicals included spray of capsicum juice, kerosene (despite its phytotoxicity) and detergents. Parasitism of aphids by *Aphidius* species and predation by coccinellid larvae and adults was high but they came late long after damage was inflicted to the crop. The series of studies carried out over the years helped to determine the status of the pest in the area and point out some of the environmentally safe management options. Planting susceptible legumes may have to be limited to places where the aphid is not endemic or better use aphid-specific pesticides (such as pirimicarb). Spraying alternate hosts during the off-season to break the cycle of infestation, determining the rate and frequency of botanicals such as capsicum, and ensuring the survival of coccinellids and aphid parasitoids during the offseason can be the next research agenda.

In: *Pisum sativum*
Editor: Shannell Becket
ISBN: 978-1-63463-230-0

Chapter 1

REGULATION OF Fe DEFICIENCY RESPONSES IN WT PEA AND SOME OF ITS MUTANTS (*BRZ* AND *DGL*)

Francisco Javier Romera[1]*, Carlos Lucena[1], María José García[2], Esteban Alcántara[1] and Rafael Pérez-Vicente[2]

[1]Department of Agronomy. Edificio Celestino Mutis (C-4), Campus of Rabanales, University of Córdoba, Córdoba, Spain

[2]Department of Botany, Ecology and Plant Physiology. Edificio Celestino Mutis (C-4), Campus of Rabanales, University of Córdoba, Córdoba, Spain

ABSTRACT

Iron (Fe) participates in many essential plant functions, such as photosynthesis, respiration and nitrogen metabolism, including nodulation of legume plants. It is abundant in most soils but its availability is low, especially in calcareous soils (more than 30% of arable soils), where its solubility is very low and is frequent the incidence of Fe chlorosis. In these soils, one of the more important factors causing Fe chlorosis is bicarbonate while hypoxia, due to flooding or other causes, can aggravate its negative effects. According to the World Health Organization, the most common nutritional disorder in humans is Fe

* Email: ag1roruf@uco.es

deficiency, with over 30% of the world's population affected. To solve both problems, two of the main objectives of plant Fe researchers are to obtain genotypes more efficient in Fe uptake (more tolerant to calcareous soils) and to get edible seeds with higher Fe content for human nutrition. For these goals, it is necessary to know better the mechanisms implicated in Fe uptake and their regulation. To acquire Fe from soils, plants have developed different strategies. Today, two main strategies are considered: the Strategy I, present in non graminaceous plants (dicots, non grasses monocots,...) and the Strategy II, present in graminaceous plants. When plants suffer from Fe deficiency they switch on several morphological and physiological changes in their roots, known as Fe deficiency stress responses (hereafter named Fe responses), aimed to facilitate Fe acquisition and mobilization. These responses are switched off once plants acquire enough Fe, to avoid Fe intoxication and energy lost. Since pea is a dicot plant species, this review is devoted to describe the characteristics of Fe acquisition and Fe responses in Strategy I plants, pointing out the role of some pea mutants (*brz* and *dgl*) in the studies about this Strategy.

Keywords: bronze mutant, chlorosis, dgl mutant, ethylene, iron, regulation, iron responses

INTRODUCTION

Iron (Fe) participates in many essential plant functions, such as photosynthesis, respiration and nitrogen metabolism [1-2]. In most cases, Fe is involved in the transport of electrons and participates as co-factor of numerous enzymes [2]. In relation to legume crops, such as pea, Fe plays a very important role in the nodulation process since it is required for some of the proteins implicated: leghemoglobin, nitrogenase, cytochromes,... [3]. Fe is abundant in most soils but its availability is low, especially in calcareous soils (more than 30% of arable soils), where its solubility is very low and is frequent the incidence of Fe chlorosis [4]. In these soils, one of the more important factors causing Fe chlorosis is bicarbonate while hypoxia, due to flooding or other causes, can aggravate its negative effects [5]. According to the World Health Organization, the most common nutritional disorder in humans is Fe deficiency, with over 30% of the world's population affected [6]. Among the plant species frequently affected by Fe chlorosis are several legume crops, such as bean, soybean, peanut, pea and others [7]. The usual way to correct Fe deficiency is the application to soil of Fe chelates, which are very expensive and easily lixiviated to the environment, that can become contaminated. In the long term, the best way to correct this deficiency is the prevention by using tolerant genotypes and adequate crop management techniques. In the case of pea, although Fe chlorosis is a worldwide agricultural problem in this species, variability in tolerance exists among different pea genotypes [8-13]. Accordingly, a number of pea breeding programmes around the world have conducted screens for variation in Fe deficiency tolerance and found significant variation for this trait. To further improve the obtention of Fe chlorosis tolerant varieties, it is necessary to know better which are the mechanisms involved in Fe acquisition and how are regulated by plants.

To facilitate Fe acquisition, plants have developed different strategies. Based on them, plants are classified in two categories: Strategy I plants, that include non grasses plants, and Strategy II plants, that include the grasses [1,14]. Strategy II plants favor the acquisition of Fe by releasing Fe^{3+} chelating agents (phytosiderophores) to soils (for recent information about Strategy II plants, the reader is referred to [1]). Since pea belongs to the Strategy I plants, we will describe Strategy I in more detail (see Fe acquisition in…).

Under Fe-deficient conditions, Strategy I plants induce morphological and physiological changes in their roots, known as Fe responses, which favor Fe acquisition. These responses are induced under Fe deficiency and are shut down once plants acquire sufficient Fe, to avoid excess Fe accumulation and energy lost. Their regulation is not totally known but in the last years evidence has been accumulating suggesting that different hormones [ethylene, auxin and nitric oxide (NO)] are involved in their activation while some Fe-related signals, probably coming from shoots to roots through the phloem, would act as inhibitors (see Regulation of Fe responses…).

In the study of the regulation of Fe responses in Strategy I plants is important the use of two pea mutants with altered regulation of these responses: *brz* (*bronze*) and *dgl*. Both mutants present constitutive activation of Fe responses even when grown under Fe-sufficient conditions [15-19]. Consequently, both hyperaccumulate Fe in their vegetative tissues when grown under Fe-sufficient conditions and can become intoxicated [17,19-20]. The genes related to the *brz* and *dgl* mutations have not been identified yet but the research aimed to decipher them can open the way to a better knowledge of the regulation of Fe acquisition in dicot plants (see Use of pea mutants…). This knowledge would allow the obtention of more Fe-efficient genotypes and seeds with higher Fe content.

The study of the regulation of Fe responses by using these pea mutants (and other approaches) is not solely important in relation to Fe nutrition but also in relation to other aspects related to plant nutrition and nodulation. As examples, it should be mentioned that these mutants are also affected in the accumulation of Al [21] and other micronutrients besides Fe [17], and also in nodulation [20, 22].

FE ACQUISITION IN DICOT PLANTS

The main characteristic of Strategy I plants, that include dicot plants such as pea and other legume crops, is the necessity of reducing Fe^{3+}, the most abundant in soils, to Fe^{2+}, which is the one preferentially absorbed. The Fe^{3+} reduction is mediated by a ferric reductase while the Fe^{2+} uptake is mediated by a Fe^{2+} transporter, both of them located in the plasma membrane of root epidermal cells [1]. The genes encoding the ferric reductase and the Fe^{2+} transporter were first cloned in Arabidopsis (*AtFRO2*, Ferric Reductase Oxidase [23]; *AtIRT1*, Iron Regulated Transporter [24]), and subsequent homologs have been cloned in other plant species, such as tomato and cucumber [25-27]. In pea, the gene encoding the ferric reductase (*PsFRO1*) was cloned by Waters et al [28] and the gene encoding the Fe^{2+} transporter (*PsRIT1*, Root Iron Transporter) by Cohen et al [29]. The ferric reductase has also been cloned in other legume crops, such as peanut (*AhFRO1* [30]) and *Medicago truncatula* (*MtFRO1* [31]). The enhanced expression of *PsRIT1* (and other *IRT1*-like genes) under Fe deficiency is associated with increased uptake capacity of several divalent metals besides Fe^{2+}, like Cd^{2+}, Zn^{2+} and Mn^{2+}, which suggests that the PsRIT1 transporter (and other IRT1-like transporters) has a broad substrate range [29,32-33]. Under Fe-deficient conditions, Strategy I plants induce morphological and physiological changes in their roots, known as Fe responses, which favor Fe acquisition. Among the physiological responses are: enhanced ferric reductase activity (due to higher expression of the *FRO* gene); enhanced Fe^{2+} uptake capacity (due to higher expression of the *IRT* gene); acidification of the rhizosphere [due to higher expression of *HA* (H^+-ATPase) genes]; release of riboflavin and phenolic compounds; and enhanced production of organic acids, like citric acid [1,14]. Some H^+-ATPase genes up-regulated by Fe deficiency are already known in dicot plants, such as the *CsHA1* in cucumber [27,34]. To our knowledge, no H^+-ATPase gene related to Fe deficiency has been identified in pea yet although it has been cloned in the legume *Medicago truncatula* (*MtHA1* [31]). Among the morphological responses are: development of root hairs and transfer cells [1,14]. Both physiological and morphological responses are located in the subapical regions of the roots [14,34]. The morphological responses are rarely mentioned in the studies about Fe in pea because root hairs are not as prominent as in other plant species and transfer cells have not been studied yet in this plant species (at least, to our knowledge).

The Fe responses are induced under Fe deficiency and are shut down once plants acquire sufficient Fe, to avoid excess Fe accumulation and energy lost. Their regulation is not totally known but in the last years evidence has been accumulating suggesting that ethylene [and other hormones such as auxin and nitric oxide (NO)] could be involved in their activation while some other Fe-related signals, probably coming from shoots to roots through the phloem, could act as inhibitors ([35]; see Regulation of Fe responses…).

REGULATION OF FE RESPONSES IN DICOT PLANTS

The responses of dicot plants to Fe deficiency are switched on or off depending on the Fe necessities of the plant. Their regulation is crucial for plants for, at least, two reasons. First, intracellular Fe excess can cause oxidative damage to cells because free ionic Fe catalyses the generation of hydroxyl radicals trough the Fenton reaction [36-37]. Second, the activation of Fe responses requires a lot of energy and, consequently, plants do not activate them at least the responses are strictly necessary. In the last years, the knowledge of the mechanisms involved in Fe acquisition by Strategy I plants, as well as their regulation, has increased considerably. Now, it is known that many Fe acquisition genes, that facilitate Fe uptake, are induced by Fe deficiency in roots. Moreover, some of them [such as *FRO* (reductase), *IRT* (Fe transporter) and *HA* (acidification) genes] are activated by bHLH TFs (Transcription Factors), induced themselves by Fe deficiency too [1,38]. From these bHLH TFs, FER (Fe-Efficiency Response) in tomato and its homolog FIT in Arabidopsis (bHLH29, FER-LIKE IRON DEFICIENCY INDUCED TRANSCRIPTION FACTOR; formerly named FRU or FIT1 [39]) are considered the master regulators of Fe acquisition from the medium, since their knock-out mutants are very chlorotic and lack the ability to activate most Fe responses in roots [40-43]. Other bHLH TFs involved in Fe acquisition in Arabidopsis are bHLH38, bHLH39, bHLH100 and bHLH101, which seem to be redundant and need to interact with FIT for most of their functions [44-45]. All these bHLH TFs are induced in both shoots and roots under Fe deficiency except FIT, which is solely induced in roots [38]. To our knowledge, no homologs of these bHLH TFs have been identified in pea yet.

The regulation of the morphological Fe responses by Strategy I plants is not totally known but there is evidence suggesting that the plant hormones ethylene, auxin and NO are involved in their activation [14,46-47]. In relation to the regulation of the physiological Fe responses, in the last years physiological and molecular evidence has been accumulating suggesting a key role for the plant hormone ethylene (in conjunction with other hormones, such as auxin and NO) as activator of the expression of the master regulator FER (and FIT) and, consequently, of most of the Fe acquisition genes, while some signal related to phloem Fe would act to repress their expression [34-35,48-49]. In a very recent review [35], a model for the regulation of physiological Fe responses in dicots has been proposed, that integrate both positive signals (such as ethylene, auxin, and NO) and negative signals (such as Fe coming from shoots to roots through the phloem).

In the study of the regulation of Fe responses by Strategy I plants, it has been very important the use of mutants with altered regulation of these responses, such as the pea *brz* and *dgl* mutants (see Use of mutants…).

USE OF MUTANTS TO STUDY REGULATION: PEA *BRZ* AND *DGL*

Despite the involvement of ethylene and phloem Fe in the regulation of physiological Fe responses by Strategy I plants, there are still many questions to solve. As examples, it is necessary to clarify which is exactly the Fe-related compound moving in the phloem that acts as repressive signal of Fe responses in roots. Additionally, it is also necessary to know how interacts this Fe-related compound with ethylene (and other hormones, such as NO) in the roots.

For the study of the regulation of Fe responses, the use of mutants has been, and will be, fundamental. We can classify the mutants employed in two main categories: hormonal mutants and mutants altered in the regulation of Fe responses. Hormonal mutants are mutants altered in the production or perception of a particular hormone, and have been used to analyze the participation of hormones in the regulation of Fe responses. During the last years, Fe researchers have used mutants related to several hormones but most of the works have been done with ethylene mutants: ethylene insensitive mutants (Arabidopsis *etr1*, *ein2* and *ein3eil1*,…; *Medicago truncatula sickle*; Soybean *etr1*), ethylene constitutive mutants (Arabidopsis *ctr1*) and ethylene overproducer mutants (Arabidopsis *eto*) [5,14,34,47,50-52]. The use of ethylene insensitive mutants has served to demonstrate that ethylene is involved in the development of subapical root hairs (reviewed in [14]) and other Fe responses [52].

The mutants altered in the regulation of Fe responses can be divided in two types: mutants that can not activate Fe responses under Fe deficiency and mutants that constitutively activate them even when grown under Fe sufficiency. Among the first ones, we can mention the tomato *fer* mutant and the Arabidopsis *fit* mutant, affected in the FER (or its homolog FIT) TF. These knock-out mutants are very chlorotic and lack the ability to activate most Fe responses in roots [40-43]. Other mutant of similar characteristics is the melon *fefe* mutant, that is probably affected in some step upstream of the melon FER homolog [53]. The study of the *fer* mutant has allowed the identification of the master regulator FER [41] and, later on, of its homolog FIT [42-43].

Among the mutants that show constitutive activation of Fe responses, even when grown under Fe-sufficient conditions, we can mention the Arabidopsis *frd3*, *opt3-2* and *nas4x* mutants; the tomato *chloronerva* mutant; and the pea *brz* (also named E107) and *dgl* mutants [15-20,49,54-57]. Most of these mutants are related, either directly or indirectly, with the movement of Fe in the phloem. Arabidopsis *frd3* (*ferric reductase defective*) is impaired in the movement of Fe in the xylem but, because this, less Fe goes to leaves (this mutant is chlorotic) and, consequently, less Fe can recirculate back from leaves to roots through the phloem [34]. In supporting this view, it should be mentioned that Fe responses are repressed in this mutant when is sprayed with Fe in its leaves [34, 49]. Arabidopsis *opt3-2* (*oligopeptide transporter*) is affected in phloem Fe because OPT3 is presumably a transporter involved in the loading of Fe into the phloem [56,58]. Arabidopsis *nas4x* (*nicotianamine synthase*) and tomato *chloronerva* mutants are also related to phloem Fe since these mutants are defective in the synthesis of NA (nicotianamine: non proteinogenic aminoacid), a chelating agent implied in the movement of Fe (and other metals) within the plant and in the unloading of Fe out of the phloem [54,57,59]. For the pea *dgl* mutant there are also some evidence suggesting that it is impaired in the movement of a Fe-related signal in the phloem [18,49,60; see below].

To date, it is not known which genes are affected in the pea *brz* and *dgl* mutants although there have been several studies about them that we are going to comment in the following paragraphs.

The pea *brz* mutant (also named E107) was the result of mutagenesis with ethylmethane sulfonic acid of the *Pisum sativum* (L.) cv 'Sparkle' [20]. The *brz* mutant phenotype is under monogenic semidominant control and has several pleiotropic effects: decreased nodulation, altered Fe responses and increased Al uptake [15-17,20-22]. The pea *dgl* mutant is an X-ray induced mutant line of *Pisum sativum* (L.) cv 'Dippes Gelbe Viktoria' or 'DGV' [61]. There is also a near isogenic line homozygous for the *dgl* mutation from the wt cv 'Sparkle' [Sparkle (*dgl*, *dgl*)] [60], that allow better comparative studies among the wt cv 'Sparkle' and its mutants: *dgl* [Sparkle (*dgl*, *dgl*)] and *brz* [Sparkle (*brz*, *brz*)]. The *dgl* mutant phenotype is also under monogenic semidominant control and has similar pleiotropic effects to the *brz* mutant: decreased nodulation and altered Fe responses [18,20]. The two genes partially complement one another, indicating that *brz* and *dgl* are not allelic but that can interact physiologically [20].

Both pea mutants (*brz* and *dgl*) present constitutive activation of Fe responses when grown under Fe-sufficient conditions: enhanced ferric reductase activity, enhanced capacity for Fe^{2+} uptake and acidification of the medium [15-19]. The two first responses can be explained by the constitutive activation of the *PsFRO1* and *PsRIT1* genes under Fe-sufficient conditions (Figure 1;[28]). As a consequence of the constitutive activation of Fe responses, both mutants hyperaccumulate Fe in their vegetative tissues when grown under Fe-sufficient conditions and can become intoxicated (Figure 2;[17,19-20]). In fact, the name *brz* (*<u>br</u>on<u>z</u>e*) derives from the bronze color of the necrotic leaf spots caused by Fe excess in the leaves of this mutant [20]. Similarly, the name *dgl* comes from <u>d</u>e<u>g</u>enerated <u>l</u>eaflets (Figure 2;[36,61]). Besides Fe, the *brz* mutant also accumulates other metals in shoots, such as Zn, Mn and Al [17,21]. As a consequence of the Fe hyperaccumulation in the *brz* and *dgl* mutants, both of them also accumulate ferritin in leaves [36] and NA in leaves and roots [37] to very high levels. Ferritins are proteins with high capacity for Fe storage and act as a buffer for this element, protecting cells from harmful concentration of free Fe [62]. NA is a chelating agent for Fe and other metals, that has been involved in their movement within the plant [57,59] and also in Fe detoxification [37].

Reciprocal grafting experiments between wt cultivars and each of these mutants have been done to know whether the *BRZ* and *DGL* genes are associated with either roots or shoots. In the case of *brz*, the results obtained with this approach have been contradictory. Welch and LaRue [17] grafted the wt cv 'Sparkle'(Sp) onto *brz* roots (Sp/*brz*) and vice versa (*brz*/Sp), and found that Fe accumulation in leaves only occurred when the *brz* genotype acted as roots (Sp/*brz*). This clearly indicates that the *brz* mutation is related to roots [17]. However, some years later Grusak and Pezeshgi [18] did similar experiments and found that enhanced ferric reductase activity was higher in the *brz*/Sp combination than in the Sp/*brz* one, which suggests that the *brz* mutation is related to shoots. We think this needs further clarification. In relation to the *dgl* mutation, Grusak and Pezeshgi [18] showed, by grafting *dgl* onto its wild type DGV (*dgl*/DGV), that the ferric reductase activity of the grafted plants was up-regulated in relation to the DGV/DGV combination, which suggests that the *dgl* mutation is related to shoots. The authors explained the above results by suggesting that the *dgl* shoots transmit a signal compound that acts as a promoter of Fe responses in the DGV roots [18]. Now, these results can also be explained by considering that the *dgl* mutant is impaired in the movement of a Fe-related repressive signal from leaves to roots through the phloem: when the *dgl* mutant is sprayed with Fe in its leaves, the Fe responses are not repressed as occurred in the wt cultivar 'Sparkle' [49].

In addition to the experiments trying to associate the *brz* and *dgl* mutations with either roots or shoots, there are also some experimental results showing that both mutants have alterations related, either directly or indirectly, to ethylene, the plant hormone that plays a key role in the activation of Fe

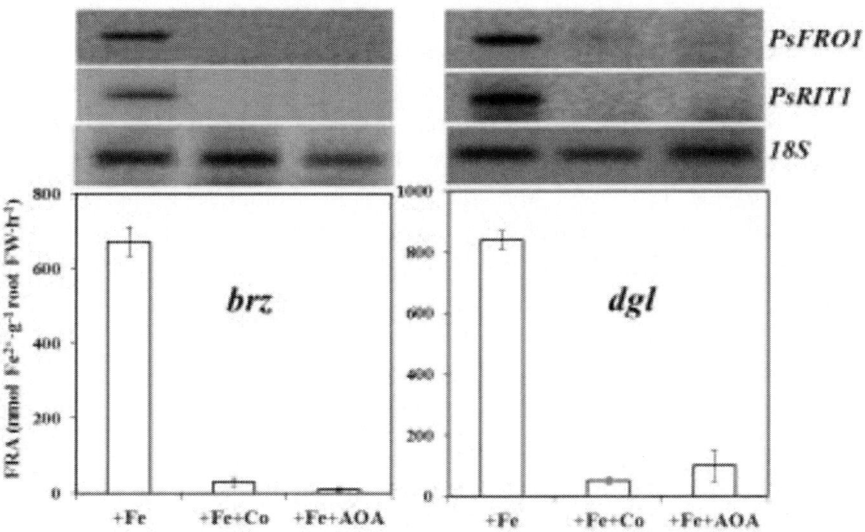

Figure 1. Effects of the ethylene inhibitors Co (cobalt) and AOA (amino-oxyacetic acid) on the expression of the Fe acquisition genes *PsFRO1* and *PsRIT1* and on the ferric reductase activity (FRA) in roots of the pea *brz* and *dgl* mutants. Plants (16-d-old) were grown in nutrient solution with 3 μM Fe-EDDHA. $CoSO_4$ (10 μM) or AOA (20 μM) was applied to some of the plants during the last 24h. FRA and gene expression were determined as in [5].

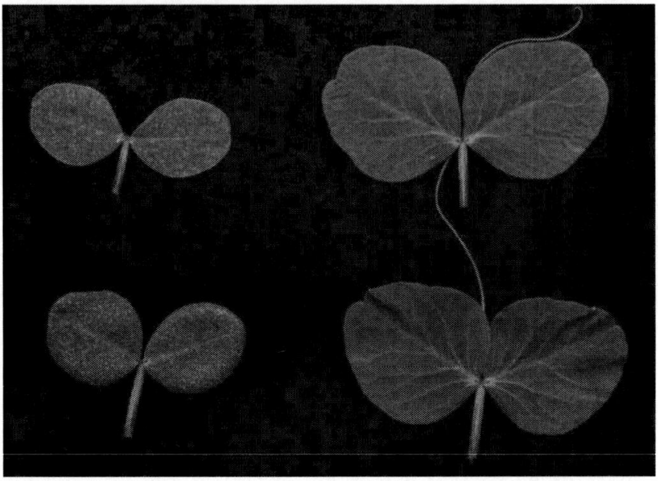

Figure 2. Fe toxicity symptoms in leaves of the pea *dgl* mutant when grown in nutrient solution with 10 μM Fe-EDDHA (left). For comparison, leaves of the wt cv 'Sparkle' grown under the same conditions (right). Notice the necrotic spots in the *dgl* leaves. To avoid this toxicity, both mutants, *dgl* and *brz*, should be cultivated in nutrient solution with 2-3 μM Fe-EDDHA.

responses (see Regulation of Fe responses…). In both mutants, their enhanced ferric reductase activity and their constitutive activation of the Fe acquisition genes *PsFRO1* and *PsRIT1* are inhibited upon addition of ethylene inhibitors to the medium (Figure 1;[19]). Moreover, the *brz* mutant exhibits a low root nodulation ability [20], which is partly restored upon treatment with the ethylene inhibitors AVG or Ag^+ [22]. The *dgl* mutant also exhibits a low root nodulation ability [20]. Since ethylene inhibits root nodulation [63], it is tempting to suggest that both mutants could have some alterations related to ethylene metabolism or perception [19].

ADAPTATION OF PEA TO IRON CHLOROSIS

Iron deficiency has been reported for many plant species and geographical regions. The most common problems occur in sensitive crops cultivated in arid and semi-arid regions, where calcareous soils are abundant [7]. In these soils, bicarbonate is one of the most important factors causing Fe chlorosis in dicot plants while hypoxia can aggravate its negative effects [5]. Factors that increase bicarbonate concentration and/or that cause hypoxia in soils, like high moisture (due to flooding or excessive irrigation) and compaction, can induce Fe chlorosis

[5]. However, the bicarbonate mode of action is not well understood. Some of its effects have been related to its pH buffering capacity (bicarbonate can maintain a high pH in the medium, which can diminish Fe solubility and Fe^{3+} reduction) but, besides these pH-mediated effects, bicarbonate can also inhibit the induction of Fe responses [5].

Fe deficiency is widely reported in several legume crops, like soybean, peanut and dry bean. Field pea is reported as a moderately sensitive crop [7], although Fe chlorosis is a worldwide agricultural problem in this species, as indicated by research works in different countries [8-13]. Most of these research works are aimed to study the variability in tolerance to calcareous soils among different pea genotypes and the physiological mechanisms behind the tolerance [8-13].

For the screening of pea genotypes tolerant to calcareous soils, several methodological approaches are employed, similar to the ones used for other dicot plants. The most direct one is to compare the behaviour of different genotypes when grown in calcareous soils, either in pots or in the field [11]. Another common approach is to compare the genotypes when grown in nutrient solution with bicarbonate, that simulate the conditions of calcareous soils [8-13]. For pea, the bicarbonate concentrations more frequently used ranged from 10 to 15 mM [8-13]. The parameters commonly used to compare the behaviour of the different genotypes are chlorosis score, chlorophyll content in young leaves, Fe concentration, active Fe concentration (it not the total Fe), and shoot and root growth [8-13]. It has been found that the root to shoot ratio increases upon bicarbonate treatment, and some authors have tried to relate this parameter to the tolerance (frequently, sensitive cultivars have higher root to shoot ratios under bicarbonate treatment than the tolerant ones [8]) but other ones have not found such a relationship [11]. Finally, an approach that could be more frequently used in the future is the identification of physiological traits related to the tolerance to Fe deficiency. Some traits that can be used in pea to discriminate between tolerant and sensitive genotypes are the following ones. First, traits associated with Fe acquisition by roots, such as acidification capacity and capacity to enhance ferric reductase activity [9,12]. One of the problems with these traits is that they should be determined several times because they change daily [11-12]. In the case of the ferric reductase activity, some works have found a relationship with the tolerance to chlorosis but some others have not [11-12]. Other possible traits for screening are the ones related to Fe translocation from roots to shoots, such as citrate concentration, and to Fe signaling, such as ethylene production [12-13]. Finally, some authors have found that the tolerant cultivars have greater ability to enhance the antioxidant responses (Fe deficiency causes oxidative stress) at the root level upon bicarbonate treatment than the sensitive ones. Consequently, this ability could be used as a marker to select tolerant cultivars [64].

To further improve the obtention of Fe chlorosis tolerant varieties, it is necessary to know better which are the mechanisms involved in Fe acquisition and how are regulated by plants. In this way, to decipher the *BRZ* and *DGL* genes could contribute to obtain pea cultivars with more efficient Fe responses and better adapted to calcareous soils but without the problems of Fe intoxication caused by the mutations of these genes.

Iron Biofortification in Pea

According to the World Health Organization, the most common nutritional disorder in humans is Fe deficiency induced anemia, with over one-third of the world's population affected [6]. To solve this problem, a promising possibility is to obtain edible seeds with higher Fe content for human nutrition. Until now, most efforts about Fe biofortification have been focused on rice [65] but legume crops also offer interesting possibilities for, at least, two reasons. First, they are an important source of nutrients for humans, especially in parts of the developing world [66]. Second, seeds of legumes, such as pea, normally have higher Fe concentrations than cereal grains and other edible vegetables [6,67]. Moreover, there is a great variability in seed Fe among different pea cultivars, ranging from 23 to 105 $mgKg^{-1}$ [67], which can be used in breeding programs.

The amount of Fe in the seeds depends on uptake from the soil into the roots, translocation into the shoots via the xylem, transfer into the leaves and other structures and translocation into the seeds via the phloem [65-66,68]. Iron content decreased in the vegetative tissues of pea plants during the reproductive phase indicating remobilization of Fe from leaves to seeds. However, continued Fe uptake and transport during seed fill is as important as remobilization [66].

To get seeds with higher Fe content (Fe biofortification) different strategies can be used, besides the traditional breeding programs. A first strategy is to increase uptake of Fe from the soils: i.e., by overexpressing ferric reductase or iron transporter genes [65]. As example, Vasconcelos et al [69] have overexpressed the *AtFRO2* gene in soybean. The transgenic lines obtained accumulate higher Fe levels in leaves than the wt ones but similar seed Fe concentrations, which suggests that the increase of Fe uptake alone is not enough. This is logical since Fe moves to leaves via xylem but to seeds it moves mainly via phloem, as xylem flow is driven by transpiration and seeds almost do no transpire. A second strategy is to "pull" Fe into the plant by increasing the sink strength: i.e., by overexpressing Fe storage ferritin genes [68]. A third strategy is to increase Fe mobilization within the plant: i.e., by increasing transporters or substrates of transporters, like *YSL* genes (involved in NA-Fe transport) or *NAS* genes (involved in NA synthesis) [2,65,68]. Most frequently, Fe researchers use a combination of several of these strategies to obtain seeds with higher Fe content [65,68].

The obtention of seeds with high Fe content is not enough for human nutrition: Fe in seeds should be bioavailable. For this, it is important the nature of the Fe compounds in seeds, the location of Fe within the seed and the presence of substances that negatively interact with Fe bioavailability, like phytic acid [65]. The location of Fe within the seeds is important in some plant species, such as rice, where Fe accumulates in external tissues discarded during processing and Fe content is very low in the endosperm [2]. In pea seeds, Fe is accumulated in the epidermis of embryos [2]. Some approaches used to increase Fe bioavailability in seeds are the use of endosperm-specific promoters to locate Fe in rice endosperm and the use of phytase genes to diminish phytic acid in seeds [2,65].

In relation to the Fe biofortification of pea, to our knowledge none of the strategies mentioned in the previous paragraphs have been applied to this plant species yet. Nonetheless, there are studies related to this topic, most of them carried out with the *brz* and *dgl* mutants, that could be very useful for pea Fe biofortification in the future. As previously mentioned (see Use of mutants…), both mutants present constitutive activation of Fe responses and, as consequence, both hyperaccumulate Fe in leaves. For comparison, while the wt pea 'Sparkle' and 'DGV' accumulate Fe around 100 µg/g DW in leaves, *brz* and *dgl* can accumulate 5000 to 10000 µg/g DW [6,20]. Since both genes function in a semi-dominant manner, F_1 hybrids exhibit intermediate leaf Fe concentrations [6,20]. Despite the *brz* mutant accumulates high levels of Fe in leaves, no increase was measured in the Fe concentration of seeds [6], with suggests that the remobilization from leaves to seeds through the phloem is similar to the wt. In supporting this view, both *brz* and its wt parent (cv 'Sparkle'), when grown with sufficient or excess Fe, exhibit seed Fe concentrations of 70 to 80 µg/g DW [6]. However, for the *dgl* mutant the results are different. When grown with sufficient or excess Fe, Fe concentration in *dgl* seeds was 250 µg/g DW, 3.5-fold that of wt seeds [6]. These results suggest that the *dgl* mutation is related to some alteration in the movement of Fe through the phloem [6,18,49,60; see Use of mutants…). This paves the way to get pea seeds with higher Fe content once the *DGL*, and its function, can be deciphered. The knowledge and adequate manipulation of the DGL function could allow the obtention of high-Fe pea seeds but without the Fe toxicity problems caused by the *dgl* mutation.

CONCLUSION

The research aimed to decipher the *brz* and *dgl* mutations can open the way to obtain pea cultivars more tolerant to calcareous soils and to get pea seeds with higher Fe content. The knowledge obtained with these mutants could also be applied to other plant species. The study of the regulation of Fe deficiency responses by using these pea mutants (and other approaches) is not solely important in relation to Fe nutrition but also in relation to other aspects related to plant mineral nutrition and to nodulation. As examples, it should be mentioned that these mutants are also affected in the nodulation process and in the accumulation of other elements besides Fe, such as the micronutrients Zn and Mn, and the toxic element Al.

REFERENCES

[1] Kobayashi, T. & Nishizawa, N.K. (2012). Iron uptake, translocation and regulation in higher plants. *Ann. Rev. Plant Biol*, *63*, 131-152.

[2] Grillet, L., Mari, S. & Schmidt, W. (2014). Iron in seeds–loading pathways and subcellular localization. *Front. Plant Sci.*, *4*, 535. doi:10.3389/ fpls.2013.00535

[3] Brear, E.M., Day, D.A. & Smith, P.M.C. (2013). Iron: an essential micronutrient for the legume–rhizobium symbiosis. *Front. Plant Sci.*, *4*, 359. doi:10.3389/ fpls.2013.00359

[4] Lindsay, W.L. (1995). Chemical reactions in soils that affect iron availability to plants. A quantitative approach. In J. Abadía J (Ed.), *Iron nutrition in soils and plants* (pp. 7-14). Dordrecht, The Netherlands: Kluwer Academic Publishers.

[5] García, M.J., García-Mateo, M.J., Lucena C., Romera, F.J., Rojas, C.L., Alcántara, E. & Pérez-Vicente, R. (2014). Hypoxia and bicarbonate

could block the expression of iron acquisition genes in Strategy I plants by affecting ethylene synthesis and signalling in different ways. *Physiol Plant.*, *150*, 95–106.

[6] Grusak, M.A. (2000). Strategies for improving the iron nutritional quality of seed crops: lessons learned from the study of unique iron-hyperaccumulating pea mutants. *Pisum Genet.*, *32*, 1-5.

[7] Hansen, N.C., Hopkins, B.G., Ellsworth, J.W. & Jolley, V.D. (2007). Iron nutrition in field crops. In L.L. Barton & J. Abadía (Eds.), *Iron nutrition in plants and rhizospheric microorganisms* (pp. 23-59). Dordrecht, The Netherlands: Springer.

[8] Zribi, K. & Gharsalli, M. (2002). Effect of bicarbonate on growth and iron nutrition of pea. *J. Plant Nutr.*, *25*, 2143-2149.

[9] Jelali, N., Wissal, M., Dell'Orto, M., Abdelly, C., Gharsalli, M. & Zocchi, G. (2010). Changes of metabolic responses to direct and induced Fe deficiency of two *Pisum sativum* cultivars. *Environ. Exp. Bot.*, *68*, 238–246.

[10] Jelali, N., Ben Salah, I., Wissal, M., Donnini, S., Zocchi, G. & Gharsalli, M. (2011). Comparison of three pea cultivars (*Pisum sativum*) regarding their responses to direct and bicarbonate-induced iron deficiency. *Sci. Hort.*, *129*, 548–553

[11] Yakop, U.M. (2012). Physiological and genetic investigations of iron deficiency in field peas (*Pisum sativum* L.). *Ph. D. Thesis*, University of Adelaide, Australia.

[12] Kabir, A.H., Paltridge, N.G., Able, A.J., Paull, J.G. & Stangoulis, J.C.R. (2012). Natural variation for Fe-efficiency is associated with up-regulation of Strategy I mechanisms and enhanced citrate and ethylene synthesis in *Pisum sativum* L. *Planta*, *235*, 1409–1419.

[13] Kabir, A.H., Paltridge, N.G., Roessner, U. & Stangoulis, J.C.R. (2013). Mechanisms associated with Fe-deficiency tolerance and signaling in shoots of *Pisum sativum*. *Physiol Plant.*, *147*, 381–395.

[14] Romera, F.J. & Alcántara, E. (2004). Ethylene involvement in the regulation of Fe-deficiency stress responses by Strategy I plants. *Funct. Plant Biol.*, *31*, 315-328.

[15] Grusak, M.A., Kochian, L.V. & Welch R.M. (1990). A transport mutant of pea (*Pisum sativum*) for the study of iron absorption in higher plant roots. In M.L. van Beusichem (Ed.), *Plant nutrition –physiology and applications* (pp. 219-22). Dordrecht, The Netherlands: Kluwer Academic Publishers.

[16] Grusak, M.A., Welch, R.M. & Kochian, L.V. (1990). Physiological characterization of a single-gene mutant of *Pisum sativum* exhibiting excess iron accumulation. *Plant Physiol.*, *93*, 976-981.
[17] Welch, R.M. & LaRue, T.A. (1990). Physiological characteristics of Fe accumulation in the 'Bronze' mutant of *Pisum sativum* L., cv 'Sparkle' E107 (*brz brz*). *Plant Physiol.*, *93*, 723-729.
[18] Grusak, M.A. & Pezeshgi, S. (1996). Shoot-to-root signal transmission regulates root Fe(III) reductase in the *dgl* mutant of pea. *Plant Physiol.*, *110*, 329-334.
[19] Romera, F.J., Welch, R.M., Norvell, W.A., Schaefer, S.C. & Kochian, L.V. (1996). Ethylene involvement in the over-expression of Fe(III)-chelate reductase by roots of E107 pea [*Pisum sativum* L. (*brz,brz*)] and chloronerva tomato (*Lycopersicon esculentum* L.) mutant genotypes. *BioMetals*, *9*, 38-44.
[20] Kneen, B.E., LaRue, T.A., Welch, R.M. & Weeden, N.F. (1990). Pleiotropic effects of *brz*. A mutation in *Pisum sativum* (L.) cv 'Sparkle' conditioning decreased nodulation and increased iron uptake and leaf necrosis. *Plant Physiol.*, *93*, 717-722.
[21] Guinel, F.C. & LaRue, T.A. (1993). Excessive aluminium accumulation in the pea mutant El07 (*brz*). *Plant Soil*, *157*, 75-82, 1993.
[22] Guinel, F.C. & LaRue, T.A. (1992). Ethylene inhibitors partly restore nodulation to pea mutant E107 (*brz*). *Plant Physiol.*, *99*, 515-518.
[23] Robinson, N.J., Procter, C.M., Connolly, E.L. & Guerinot, M.L. (1999). A ferric-chelate reductase for iron uptake from soils. *Nature*, *397*, 694-697.
[24] Eide, D., Broderius, M., Fett, J. & Guerinot, M.L. (1996). A novel iron-regulated metal transporter from plants identified by functional expression in yeast. *Proc. Natl. Acad. Sci. USA*, *93*, 5624-5628.
[25] Eckhardt, U., Mas Marques, A. & Buckhout, T.J. (2001). Two iron-regulated cation transporters from tomato complement metal uptake deficient yeast. *Plant Mol. Biol.*, *45*, 437-448.
[26] Li, L., Cheng, X. & Ling, H.Q. (2004). Isolation and characterization of Fe(III)-chelate reductase gene *LeFRO1* in tomato. *Plant Mol. Biol.*, *54*, 125-136.
[27] Waters, B.M., Lucena, C., Romera, F.J., Jester, G.G., Wynn, A.N., Rojas, C.L., Alcántara, E. & Pérez-Vicente, R. (2007). Ethylene involvement in the regulation of the H^+-ATPase *CsHA1* gene and of the new isolated ferric reductase *CsFRO1* and iron trasnporter *CsIRT1* genes in cucumber plants. *Plant Physiol. Biochem.*, *45*, 293-301.

[28] Waters, B.M., Blevins, D.G. & Eide, D.J. (2002). Characterization of FRO1, a pea ferric-chelate reductase involved in root iron acquisition. *Plant Physiol.*, *129*, 85-94.

[29] Cohen, C.K., Garvin, D.F. & Kochian, L.V. (2004). Kinetic properties of a micronutrient transporter from *Pisum sativum* indicate a primary function in Fe uptake from the soil. *Planta*, *218*, 784-792.

[30] Ding, H., Duan, L., Wu, H., Yang, R., Ling, H., Li, W.X. & Zhang, F. (2009). Regulation of AhFRO1, an Fe(III)-chelate reductase of peanut, during iron deficiency stress and intercropping with maize. *Physiol. Plant.*, *136*, 274–283.

[31] Andaluz, S., Rodríguez-Celma, J., Abadía, A., Abadía, J. & López-Millán, A.F. (2009). Time course induction of several key enzymes in *Medicago truncatula* roots in response to Fe deficiency. *Plant Physiol. Biochem.*, *47*, 1082–1088

[32] Cohen, C.K., Fox, T.C., Garvin, D.F. & Kochian, L.V. (1998). The role of iron-deficiency stress responses in stimulating heavy-metal transport in plants. *Plant Physiol.*, *116*, 1063–1072.

[33] Korshunova, Y.O., Eide, D., Clark, W.G., Guerinot, M.L. & Pakrasi, H.B. (1999). The IRT1 protein from *Arabidopsis thaliana* is a metal transporter with a broad substrate range. *Plant Mol. Biol.*, *40*, 37–44.

[34] Lucena, C., Waters, B.M., Romera, F.J., García, M.J., Morales, M., Alcántara, E. & Pérez-Vicente, R. (2006). Ethylene could influence ferric reductase, iron transporter and H^+-ATPase gene expression by affecting FER (or FER-like) gene activity. *J. Exp. Bot.*, *57*, 4145-4154.

[35] Romera, F.J., Lucena, C., García, M.J., Alcántara, E. & Pérez-Vicente, R. (2014). The role of ethylene and other signals in the regulation of Fe deficiency responses by dicot plants. In M. Sarwat (Ed.), *Stress Signalling in Plants: Genomics and Proteomics Perspectives, Vol 2* (in press). New York, USA: Springer.

[36] Becker, R., Manteuffel, R., Neumann, D. & Scholz, G. (1998). Excessive iron accumulation in the pea mutants *dgl* and *brz*: subcellular localization of iron and ferritin. *Planta*, *207*, 217-223.

[37] Pich, A., Manteuffel, R., Hillmer, S., Scholz, G. & Schmidt, W. (2001). Fe homeostasis in plant cells: does nicotianamine play multiple roles in the regulation of cytoplasmic Fe concentration? *Planta*, *213*, 967-976.

[38] Wang, H.Y., Klatte, M., Jakoby, M., Bäumlein, H., Weisshaar, B. & Bauer, P. (2007). Iron deficiency-mediated stress regulation of four subgroup Ib *BHLH* genes in *Arabidopsis thaliana*. *Planta*, *226*, 897–908.

[39] Bauer, P., Ling, H.Q. & Guerinot, M.L. (2007). *FIT*, the *FER-LIKE IRON DEFICIENCY INDUCED TRANSCRIPTION FACTOR* in *Arabidopsis. Plant Physiol. Biochem.*, *45*, 260-261.
[40] Brown, J.C., Chaney, R.L. & Ambler, J.E. (1971). A new tomato mutant inefficient in the transport of iron. *Physiol. Plant.*, *25*, 48-53.
[41] Ling, H.Q., Bauer, P., Bereczky, Z., Keller, B. & Ganal, M. (2002). The tomato *fer* gene encoding a bHLH protein controls iron-uptake responses in roots. *Proc. Natl. Acad. Sci. USA*, *99*, 13938-13943.
[42] Colangelo, E.P. & Guerinot, M.L. (2004). The essential basic helix-loop-helix protein FIT1 is required for the iron deficiency response. *Plant Cell*, *16*, 3400-3412.
[43] Jakoby, M,, Wang, H.Y., Reidt, W., Weisshaar, B. & Bauer, P. (2004). *FRU* (*BHLH029*) is required for induction of iron mobilization genes in *Arabidopsis thaliana. FEBS Lett.*, *577*, 528-534.
[44] Yuan, Y.X., Wu, H.L., Wang, N., Li, J., Zhao, W.N., Du, J., Wang, D.W. & Ling, H.Q. (2008). FIT interacts with AtbHLH038 and AtbHLH039 in regulating iron uptake gene expression for iron homeostasis in *Arabidopsis. Cell. Res.*, *18*, 85-397.
[45] Wang, N., Cui, Y., Liu, Y., Fan, H., Du, J., Huang, Z, Yuan, Y., Wu, H. & Ling, H.Q. (2013). Requirement and functional redundancy of Ib subgroup bHLH proteins for iron deficiency responses and uptake in *Arabidopsis thaliana. Mol. Plant.*, *6*, 503–513.
[46] Graziano, M. & Lamattina, L. (2007). Nitric oxide accumulation is required for molecular and physiological responses to iron deficiency in tomato roots. *Plant J.*, *52*, 949-960.
[47] Romera, F.J., Lucena, C. & Alcántara, E. (2007). Plant hormones influencing iron uptake in plants. In L.L. Barton & J. Abadía (Eds.), *Iron nutrition in plants and rhizospheric microorganisms* (pp. 251-278). Dordrecht, The Netherlands: Springer.
[48] García, M.J., Suarez, V., Romera, F.J., Alcántara, E. & Pérez-Vicente, R, (2011). A new model involving ethylene, nitric oxide and Fe to explain the regulation of Fe-acquisition genes in Strategy I plants. *Plant Physiol. Biochem.*, *49*, 537-544.
[49] García, M.J., Romera, F.J., Stacey, M.G., Stacey, G., Villar, E., Alcántara, E. & Pérez-Vicente, R. (2013). Shoot to root communication is necessary to control the expression of iron-acquisition genes in Strategy I plants. *Planta*, *237*, 65-75.
[50] García, M.J., Lucena, C., Romera, F.J., Alcántara, E. & Pérez-Vicente, R. (2010). Ethylene and nitric oxide involvement in the up-regulation of

key genes related to iron acquisition and homeostasis in *Arabidopsis*. *J. Exp. Bot.*, *61*, 3885-3899.

[51] Schmidt, W., Tittel, J. & Schikora, A. (2000). Role of hormones in the induction of iron deficiency responses in Arabidopsis roots. *Plant Physiol.*, *122*, 1109-1118.

[52] Lingam, S., Mohrbacher, J., Brumbarova, T., Potuschak, T., Fink-Straube, C., Blondet, E., Genschik, P. & Bauer, P. (2011). Interaction between the bHLH transcription factor FIT and the ETHILENE INSENSITIVE3/ETHYLENE INSENSITIVE3-LIKE1 reveals molecular linkage between the regulation of iron acquisition and ethylene signaling in *Arabidopsis*. *Plant Cell*, *23*, 1815-1829.

[53] Waters, B.M., McInturf, S.A. & Amundsen, K. (2014). Transcriptomic and physiological characterization of the *fefe* mutant of melon (*Cucumis melo*) reveals new aspects of iron–copper crosstalk. *New Phytol.*, doi: 10.1111/nph.12911

[54] Ling, H.Q., Koch, G., Bäumlein, H. & Ganal, M.W. (1999). Map-based cloning of *chloronerva,* a gene involved in iron uptake of higher plants encoding nicotianamine synthase. *Proc. Natl. Acad. Sci. USA*, *96*, 7098–7103.

[55] Rogers, E.E. & Guerinot, M.L. (2002). FRD3, a member of the multidrug and toxin efflux family, controls iron deficiency responses in *Arabidopsis*. *Plant Cell*, *14*, 1787–1799.

[56] Stacey, M.G., Patel, A., McClain, W.E., Mathieu, M., Remley, M., Rogers, E.E., Gassmann, W., Blevins, D.G. & Stacey, G. (2008). The *Arabidopsis* AtOPT3 protein functions in metal homeostasis and movement of iron to developing seeds. *Plant Physiol.*, *146*, 589–601.

[57] Klatte, M., Schuler, M., Wirtz, M., Fink-Straube, C., Hell, R. & Bauer, P. (2009). The analysis of Arabidopsis nicotianamine synthase mutants reveals functions for nicotianamine in seed iron loading and iron deficiency responses. *Plant Physiol.*, *150*, 257–271.

[58] Zhai, Z., Gayomba, S.R., Jung, H.,Vimalakumari, N.K., Piñeros, M., Craft, E., Rutzke, M.A., Danku, J., Lahner, B., Punzón, T., Guerinot, M.L., Salt, D.E., Kochian, L.V. & Vatamaniuk, O.K. (2014). OPT3 is a phloem-specific iron transporter that is essential for systemic iron signaling and redistribution of iron and cadmium in *Arabidopsis*. *Plant Cell*, doi/10.1105/tpc.114.123737

[59] Schuler, M., Rellán-Álvarez, R., Fink-Straube, C., Abadía, J. & Bauer, P. (2012). Nicotianamine functions in the phloem-based transport of iron

to sink organs, in pollen development and pollen tube growth in Arabidopsis. *Plant Cell, 24*, 2380-2400.

[60] Marentes, E. & Grusak, M.A. (1998). Mass determination of low-molecular-weight proteins in phloem sap using matrix-assisted laser desorption/ionization time-of-flight mass spectrometry. *J. Exp. Bot.*, *49*, 903–911.

[61] Gottschalk, W. G. (1987). Improvement of the selection value of gene *dgl* through recombination. *Pisum Newslett*, *19*, 9-11.

[62] Lobreaux, S. & Briat, J.F. (1991). Ferritin accumulation and degradation in different organs of pea (*Pisum sativum*) during development. *Biochem. J.*, *274*, 601-606.

[63] Guinel, F.C. & Geil, R.D. (2002). A model for the development of the rhizobial and arbuscular mycorrhizal symbioses in legumes and its use to understand the roles of ethylene in the establishment of these two symbioses. *Can. J. Bot.*, *80*, 695-720.

[64] Jelali, N., Donnini, S., Dell'Orto, M., Abdelly, C., Gharsalli, M. & Zocchi, G. (2014). Root antioxidant responses of two *Pisum sativum* cultivars to direct and induced Fe deficiency. *Plant Biol.*, *16*, 607–614.

[65] Sperotto, R.A., Ricachenevsky, F.K., Waldow, V.A. & Fett, J.P. (2012). Iron biofortification in rice: It's a long way to the top. *Plant Sci.*, *190*, 24-39.

[66] Sankaran, R.P. & Grusak, M.A. (2014). Whole shoot mineral partitioning and accumulation in pea (*Pisum sativum*). *Front. Plant Sci.*, *5*, 149. doi:10.3389/fpls. 2014.00149.

[67] White, P.J. & Broadley, M. R. (2005). Biofortifyng crops with essential mineral elements. *Trends Plant Sci.*, *10*, 586-593.

[68] Waters, B.M. & Sankaran, R.P. (2011). Moving micronutrients from the soil to the seeds: Genes and physiological processes from a biofortification perspective. *Plant Sci.*, *180*, 562-574.

[69] Vasconcelos, M.W., Clemente, T.E. & Grusak, M.A. (2014). Evaluation of constitutive iron reductase (AtFRO2) expression on mineral accumulation and distribution in soybean (*Glycine max* L). *Front. Plant Sci.*, *5*, 112. doi:10.3389/fpls.2014.00112

In: *Pisum sativum*
Editor: Shannell Becket
ISBN: 978-1-63463-230-0

Chapter 2

PROTEINS AND ENZYMES OF THE PEA *PISUM SATIVUM*

Tzi Bun Ng*[*] *and Charlene Cheuk Wing Ng
School of Biomedical Sciences, Faculty of Medicine,
The Chinese University of Hong Kong,
Shatin, New Territories, Hong Kong, China

ABSTRACT

The pea *Pisum sativum* produces a diversity of enzymes and proteins. They include alpha-galactosidases, beta-galactosidase, insoluble acid invertase, germin-like protein with superoxide dismutase activity, glutathione reductase, aminoaldehyde dehydrogenase, NADP+-linked isocitrate dehydrogenase, p-aminobenzoylglutamate hydrolase, phospholipase C delta isoforms, cytoplasmic fructose-1,6-bisphosphatase, raffinose synthase, beta-ketoacyl-acyl carrier protein synthase III, caspases, DNA helicase 47, DNA helicase 45, chromatin-associated histone binding protein, beta-1,3-glucanase, symbiosis-related chitinases, Bowman-Birk protease inhibitors, angiotensin converting enzyme inhibitory peptide, antifungal proteins, C-6 oxidases, short-chain alcohol dehydrogenase-like protein, fatty acid alpha-dioxygenase, gibberellin dioxygenases, carbonic anhydrase, photosystem II proteins with carbonic anhydrase activity, C1 subgroup mitogen-activated protein kinase,

[*] Corresponding author. School of Biomedical Sciences, Faculty of Medicine, The Chinese University of Hong Kong, Shatin, New Territories, Hong Kong,China. Email : b021770@mailserv.cuhk.edu.hk.

Ca2+/calmodulin-dependent protein kinase, enzyme catalyzing conjugation of indole-3-acetic acid to aspartate, pea albumin 1F (PA1F), pea albumin 1, subunit b, vicilin, lectins, mitochondrial type II peroxiredoxin, channel-forming protein in chloroplasts, outer envelope membrane protein 16 of pea chloroplasts, cell wall fibronectin-like adhesion protein, arabinogalactan-protein-extensin glycoproteins, ferritin, and dehydrin.

Keywords: pea, *Pisum sativum*, proteins, enzymes

Introduction

Peas are rich in proteins and dietary fiber and contribute considerably to the total dietary protein requirements. Peas are abundant in complex carbohydrates giving rise to food with a low glycemic index. Peas are hypolipidemic. Fiber in peas contains more amylose than amylopectin and is antihyperglycemic. Peas can be used in processed foods such as bakery products, bread, snack foods, soups, and tortillas. Because of their nutritiousness, it has been suggested that peas be included in snack foods, baby food, and sports food (Asif et al., 2013).

The purpose of this article is to review the pea enzymes and proteins reported in the literature.

Alpha-Galactosidases

Two cDNAs encoding alpha-galactosidases from maturing and germinating pea seeds, including a member of the acidic alpha-galactosidase of the family 27 glycosyl hydrolase cluster and a member of the family of alkaline alpha-galactosidases, which display pronounced homology to seed imbibition proteins, have been isolated. Transcripts encoding the acidic alpha-galactosidase, found in protein storage vacuoles, are present in dry seeds and expressed during seed maturation and exhibit little variations in seed germination. Transcripts encoding the alkaline alpha-galactosidase are expressed after radicle protrusion (Blöch et al., 2008).

BETA-GALACTOSIDASE

A basic 55-kDa glycosylated beta-galactosidase (PsBGAL), with N-terminal sequence resemblance to its counterpart from *Arabidopsis thaliana*, has been purified from pea seeds by over 900-fold. The enzyme can hydrolyze pea seed xyloglucan, and may play a role in changing the cell wall composition in seedling growth and development. (Dwevedi and Kayastha, 2009).

INSOLUBLE ACID INVERTASE

Invertase catalyzes sucrose hydrolysis into D-glucose and D-fructose. The 69-kDa insoluble acid invertase from pea displays an isoelectric point of about pH 8.0, a pH optimum of 4.0 and a temperature optimum of 45 °C, a K(m) of 4.41 mM and a V(max) of 8.41 U (mg protein)(-1) min(-1).The enzyme has been purified by ammonium sulfate precipitation, ion exchange chromatography, absorption chromatography, reactive green-19 affinity chromatography, and gel filtration. The activity of the enzyme is unaltered by Tris-HCl and mercury chloride but inhibited by 6.2 mM copper sulfate. Its pH optimum and temperature optimum are respectively lower and higher than other invertases(Kim et al., 2011).

GERMIN-LIKE PROTEIN WITH SUPEROXIDE DISMUTASE ACTIVITY

PsGER1 is a germin-like nodule-associated pea protein with superoxide dismutase activity resistant to hydrogen peroxide, detergents, and high temperatures. PsGER1 transcript is found in expanding cells near the meristematic zone and in the epidermis. It exhibits striking sequence homology to the N-terminal sequence of a putative plant rhicadhesin (a bacterial attachment protein) receptor,. However, its location in nodules indicates functions other than a rhicadhesin receptor needed for the initial stage of bacterial attachment to root hairs (Gucciardo et al., 2007).

Glutathione Reductase

The 56-kDa glutathione reductase isozyme with an isoelectric point of 5.4 has been purified from pea leaf peroxisomes. A multiple targeting of glutathione reductase to chloroplasts, mitochondria and peroxisomes, has been observed depending on the organelle metabolism under the prevailing growth conditions.

Peroxisomal glutathione reductase plays a role in abiotic stress conditions, such as abundant light, darkness, high temperatures, low temperatures, wounding, and cadmium toxicity, (Romero-Puertas et al., 2006).

Aminoaldehyde Dehydrogenase

Aminoaldehydes are toxic polyamine breakdown products. Pea aminoaldehyde dehydrogenase was overexpressed in *E.coli*, purified and crystallized using the hanging-drop method. Crystals belong to the monoclinic space group P2(1),with unit-cell parameters a = 86.4, b = 216.6, c = 205.4 A, beta = 98.1 degrees (Tylichová et al., 2008).

NADP+-Linked Isocitrate Dehydrogenase

A homotetrameric 146-kDa NADP+-linked isocitrate dehydrogenase manifesting optimum pH at 7.5-8 and inactivation at 45-50 degrees C has been isolated from germinating pea seeds. Maximum enzyme activity is dependent on presence of Mn2+ and Mg2+ ions (3.75 mM). Activity is partially restored by addition of Ca2+, Co2+, Cd2+, and Zn2+ ions after demetallation by dialysis against EDTA and buffer (Srivastava et al., 2001).

C-6 Oxidases

C-6 oxidation genes regulate brassinosteroid activation, which involves the C-6 oxidation of 6-deoxocastasterone to castasterone (CS) and in some cases further conversion of castasterone to brassinolide (BL).

However, unlike Arabidopsis and tomato C-6 oxidases which further convert 6-deoxocastasterone to castasterone and then castasterone to brassinolide, the two pea brassinosteroid C-6 oxidases (CYP85A1 and CYP85A6) convert 6-deoxocastasterone to castasterone by C-6 oxidation (Jager et al., 2007).

SHORT-CHAIN ALCOHOL DEHYDROGENASE-LIKE PROTEIN (SAD)

The SAD gene family in pea has at least three proteins (SAD-A, SAD-B, and SAD -C). Expression of SAD-A and SAD–C in Escherichia coli or Pichia pastoris yields full-length soluble proteins. Tetrameric SAD-C protein is a dimer of dimers. Following brief exposure to ultraviolet-B radiation SAD genes are transiently expressed whereas after prolonged UV-B irradiation mRNA accumulation results in formation of SAD protein in leaves and stems (Scherbak et al., 2009).

FATTY ACID ALPHA-DIOXYGENASE

alpha-Dioxygenases catalyze the first step of the alpha-oxidation pathway of long-chain fatty acids in plants.They are expressed in plants in response to biotic and abiotic stress. During germination, alpha-dioxygenase mRNA accumulates in the cotyledons and the embryonic axis of pea seeds. In developing pea plants, the transcript is detected in roots. The accumulation of alpha-dioxygenase protein parallels transcript accumulation in that it is abundant in germinating as well as young plant tissue, and correlates with loss of mRNA during plant maturation (Meisner et al., 2009).

GIBBERELLIN DIOXYGENASES

Pea gibberellin-oxidase was expressed as a glutathione s-transferase fusion and purified with a yield of 0.3 mg/g cells by affinity chromatography, glutathione s-transferase removal and gel filtration. It displays a Km of 0.024 microM and a Vmax of 4.4 pkat/mg toward [1beta, 2beta, 3beta-3H3]GA20. Fusion tags are needed to stabilize and solubilize PsGA2OX1 during *E. coli* expression.

The availability of sizeable amounts of purified PsGA2OX1 facilitates mechanistic and structural studies (Lester et al., 2005).

Carbonic Anhydrase

Recombinant pea beta-carbonic anhydrase was purified and crystallized. Crystals belong to the orthorhombic space group C222, with unit-cell parameters a = 136.3, b = 142.5, c = 201.4 A,alpha = beta = gamma = 90 degrees. Crystals typically diffracted anisotropically,with a maximal resolution of 2.0 A in the strongest direction (Kimber et al., 2000).

Photosystem II Proteins with Carbonic Anhydrase Activity

Hydrophilic proteins of the photosystem II oxygen-evolving complex from pea leaves possess a molecular mass of 18 kDa (protein PsbQ), 24 kDa (protein PsbP), and 33 kDa (protein PsbO).They all exhibit Mn2+dependent carbonic anhydrase activity (Shitov et al., 2009).

C1 Subgroup Mitogen-Activated Protein Kinase (MAPK)

MMAPK cascades are important in plant growth and development and in responses to abiotic and biotic stress. They are classified into four major groups (A-D) based on their sequence homology. Abundant information about MAPKs in groups A and B exists but information about the C group is meager. PsMPK2 is expressed in reproductive as well as vegetative organs. Expression of pea MPK2 in Arabidopsis thaliana disclosed that mechanical injury and other stress agents as hydrogen peroxide, jasmonic acid and abscisic acid elevate the enzyme activity.Hence C1 subgroup MAPKs may play a role in the stress response (Ortiz-Masia et al., 2008)

Ca2+/Calmodulin-Dependent Protein Kinase

The 72-kDa pea Ca2+/calmodulin-dependent protein kinase activity is increased in roots at low temperatures and rising salinities. Ca2+ administration raises the kinase level more rapidly than stress application. Stress upregulation of kinase brought about by low temperatures but not by salinity is suppressed by EGTA and the calmodulin inhibitor W7 (Pandey et al., 2002).

Enzyme Catalyzing Conjugation of Indole-3-Acetic Acid to Aspartate

Enzymatic synthesis of indole-3-acetylaspartate (IAA-Asp) by a crude enzyme preparation from immature pea seeds catalyzing the conjugation of indole-3-acetic acid to aspartic acids has been reported. IAA-Asp formation is dependent on ATP and Mg2+, and was linear during a 60 min period. The optimum pH and optimum temperature of the enzyme are at pH 8.0 and at 30 degrees C, respectively (Ostrowski et al., 2008).

P-Aminobenzoylglutamate Hydrolase

p-aminobenzoylglutamate hydrolase activity, which catalyzes the hydrolysis of p-aminobenzoylglutamate and its polyglutamates to the folate biosynthesis precursor p-aminobenzoate, was observed in mitochondrial and cytosol/vacuole fractions of pea leaves (Bozzo et al., 2008).

Phospholipase C Delta Isoform

The amino acid sequence deduced from the cDNA sequence encoding a pea phospholipase C-delta exhibits substantial identity to its counterpart other plants with the typical X, Y and C2 domains. The recombinant product protein is inactive, despite possession of the requisite amino acids, although the C2 domain is capable of binding calcium. The gene is expressed in all pea tissues, and is regulated by light in a tissue-specific manner. Expression is higher in roots than in shoots (Venkataraman et al., 2003).

Cytoplasmic Fructose-1,6-Bisphosphatase

Recombinant pea cytoplasmic fructose-1,6-bisphosphatase is thermostable and active in the pH range 6.6-9.0. The activation energy is 17.4 kcal/mol, Arrhenius frequency factor is 2.6 x 10(12)/s. K(M) was 10.47 microM, and V(max) is 109 micromol/min. The recombinant enzyme is competitively inhibited by fructose-2,6-bisphosphate and non-competitively inhibited by AMP (Jang et al., 2003).

Raffinose Synthase

Steady-state kinetic analysis suggested that pea seed raffinose synthase is a transglycosidase adopting a ping-pong reaction mechanism. The activity of pea seed enzyme is markedly suppressed by 1-deoxygalactonojirimycin which inhibits alpha-galactosidases (Peterbauer et al., 2002).

Beta-Ketoacyl-Acyl Carrier Protein Synthase III

A 42-kDa dimeric beta-ketoacyl-acyl carrier protein (ACP) synthase III from pea leaves demonstrating amino acid sequence similarity to counterparts from other plants is uncompetitively inhibited by thiolactomycin but is competitively inhibited by a thiolactomycin derivative with a longer (C8 saturated) hydrophobic side-chain (compound 332) (Jones et al., 2003).

Caspases

Caspase-like proteases are important to the developmental cell death of secondary shoots of pea seedlings that appear following elimination of the epicotyl. Caspase-like activity is upregulated in aging secondary shoots, but not in dominant growing shoots, unlike papain-like cysteine protease activity which prevails in the dominant shoot. Revitalization of the aging shoot by removal of the dominant shoot causes the caspase-like activity to undergo a decline. Administration of caspase or cysteine protease inhibitors into the residual epicotyl tissue inhibits the death of the secondary shoots, generating seedlings with two equal shoots. The data reveal that shoot selection in pea seedlings is regulated by apoptosis, via the stimulation of caspase-like proteases (Belenghi et al., 2004).

DNA Helicase 47

Helicases play a role in nucleic acid metabolism and are sensitive to abiotic stresses which decrease plant growth and productivity. Induction of the transcript of pea DNA helicase 47 (PDH47) occurs in both shoots and roots under cold and salinity stress, but not drought stress. PDH47 is found in both the nucleus and cytosol. Recombinant PDH47 exhibits ATP-dependent DNA and RNA helicase and DNA-dependent ATPase activities, and 3' to 5' as well as 5' to 3' directional helicase activities. Protein kinase C phosphorylates Ser and Thr residues of PDH47 and stimulates the enzyme (Vashisht et al., 2005).

DNA Helicase 45

pea DNA helicase 45 (PDH45) shows dramatic resemblance to the eukaryotic translation initiation factor eIF-4A. Induction of PDH45 mRNA occurs in pea seedlings upon exposure to high salt. Compared with wild type plants, the T(0) transgenic plants have elevated levels of PDH45 protein under normal and stress conditions and are tolerant to high salinity. The T(1) transgenics can mature and develop normal viable seeds under salt stress without any effect on plant yield regarding seed weight. PDH45 overexpression facilitates exploitation of DNA/RNA unwinding pathways for engineering salinity tolerance without influencing crop yield (Sanan-Mishra et al., 2005).

Chromatin-Associated Histone Binding Protein

Pisum sativum p16 is a protein firmly anchored to chromatin through histones especially H3 and H4 in ungerminated embryonic axes. p16 is a nuclear protein although the protein is also present in other organelles. p16 might play a role in the changes that occur in chromatin during the processes of seed maturation and germination (Castillo et al., 2002).

Beta-1,3-Glucanase

A cDNA encoding a beta-1,3-glucanase, named PsGNS2, has been isolated. PsGNS2 expression is detected in young pea flowers and seed coat but there is low expression in roots and stems during development of the pea seedling. PsGNS2 induction is not seen following environmental stress or fungal infection (Buchner et al., 2002).

Symbiosis-Related Chitinases

A quadruple of acidic symbiosis-related 30-kDa chitinase isoforms with isoelectric points ranging between 5.2 and 5.85 has been induced after colonization of *Pisum sativum* L. cv. Frisson roots with Glomus mosseaef, an arbuscular mycorrhizal fungus. One of these isoforms sclosely resembles a pea shoot class-I chitinase isoform (Slezack et al., 2001).

Bowman-Birk Protease Inhibitors

A Bowman-Birk family of plant trypsin inhibitor (BBI) isoforms purified from pea seeds demonstrate an IC50 of 41 microM to the pea aphid *Acyrthosiphon pisum* and a LC50 of 48 microM at 7 days. Cyclic peptides with the Bowman-Birk anti-chymotrypsin head are much more toxic and growth inhibitory than the anti-trypsin counterparts. The toxicity is witnessed in restlessness of aphids fed with the toxic peptides. However, chymotrypsin activity is indiscernible in the aphid gut, and the target of the chymotrypsin inhibitor awaits elucidation (Rahbé et al., 2003).

Angiotensin Converting Enzyme (ACE) Inhibitory Peptide

Following fermentation of pea seeds by *Lactobacillus plantarum* 299v in monoculture and digestion under gastrointestinal conditions, the sequence of the ACE inhibitory peptide obtained from pea proteins has been determined and found to be DDEEEEQGEEE (Jakubczyk et al., 2013).

ANTIFUNGAL PROTEINS

Pisum sativum var. *macrocarpon* (sugar snap, also called honey pea) legumes produce sativin, a 38-kDa antifungal protein with an N-terminal sequence analogous to those of miraculin (a sweet plant protein) and pisavin (a ribosome-inactivating protein from *Pisum sativum* var. arvense Poir displaying similarity to miraculin). Sativin manifests antifungal activity against *Coprinus comatus, Fusarium oxysporum,* and *Pleurotus ostreatus* but not against *Rhizoctonia solani* (Ye et al., 2000). A31-kDa antifungal protein designated pisumin, also from the sugar snap pea, exhibits antifungal activity against *C.comatus* and *P.ostreatus* and attenuated activity against *F. oxysporum* and *R. solan*i. (Ye and Ng, 2003).

PEA ALBUMIN 1F (PA1F)

The peptide pea albumin 1F (PA1F) produces a hyperglycemic action following subcutaneous injection to normal and type II diabetic mice (KK/upj-Ay) at a dosage of 5 or 10 microg/g body weight. PA1F binding protein from murine pancreatic cell membrane, same as the voltage-dependent anion channel 1 (VDAC-1), may play a role in blood glucose regulation after PA1F binding (Dun et al., 2008).

PEA ALBUMIN 1, SUBUNIT B

PA1b (pea albumin 1, subunit b) is a cysteine-rich pea seed defense protein with 37 amino acids. It induces short-term mortality in the cereal weevils *Sitophilus granarius*, *S. oryzae*, and *S.zeamais*). The primary sequence of the protein does not share similarities with other known toxins. PA1b belongs to the inhibitor cystine-knot family with six cysteines forming three disulfide bridges. It displays a triple-stranded antiparallel beta-sheet with a long flexible loop linking the first to the second strand and a series of turns. The lipophilic and electrostatic potentials at the surface of PA1b are very close to those found in the spider toxin ACTX-Hi:OB4219, thus indicating activity on ion channels (Jouvensal et al., 2003).

VICILIN

Alkaline extraction of pea flour and salt fractionation under acid conditions have yielded two vicilin fractions, designated as vicilin 1 degrees and vicilin 2 degrees after purification. Convicilin (a band at approximately 70 kDa) is the third pea globulin found in vicilin 2 degrees (O'Kane et al., 2004).

LECTINS

Fluorescein isothiocyanate (FITC)-labelled mannose-specific lectins from two pea varieties (PG-3 and LFP-48) exert a more pronounced stimulation in homologous *Rhizobium leguminosarum* strains binding reaction although reaction with heterologous strains of *Rhizobium* spp has also been observed indicating that specificity is not very high (Bajaj et al., 2001).

A mannose- and glucose-binding lectin from sugar snap legumes is unadsorbed on Affi-gel blue gel and Q-Sepharose and adsorbed on SP-Toyopearl. The lectin shows striking homology in N-terminal sequences of its alpha- and beta-subunit to lectin from *Pisum sativum* L. var. Feltham. The only difference lied in the 19th N-terminal residue of the beta-subunit(Ye and Ng, 2001). Glucose/mannose binding *Pisum arvense* lectin is composed of two distinct polypeptide chains: alpha (Mr. 5591 Da) and beta (19986 Da) (Cavada et al., 2003).

MITOCHONDRIAL TYPE II PEROXIREDOXIN

A type II peroxiredoxin from *Pisum sativum* (estimated molecular weight 18.6 kDa) has been cloned into the pET3d vector and overexpressed in *E. coli.* The recombinant protein has been purified and crystallized by. X-ray data revealed that, with the use of hanging-drop vapour-diffusion technique, the protein crystallized in space group P1, with unit-cell parameters a = 61.88, b = 66.40, c = 77.23 angstroms, alpha = 102.90, beta = 104.40, gamma = 99.07 degrees (Barranco-Medina et al., 2006).

CHANNEL-FORMING PROTEIN IN CHLOROPLASTS

Tic110 is a channel-forming protein with six transmembrane helices with a role in the import of proteins produced in the cytosol occurring at the inner chloroplast envelope. Two N-terminal hydrophobic transmembrane helices serve as a signal for the localization of the protein to the membrane. The remaining amphipathic transmembrane helices are found in residues 92-959. Calcium ions exert a marked effect on channel activity *in vitro*. The channel-forming protein possesses a redox-active disulfide which potentially can interact with stromal thioredoxin (Balsera et al., 2009).

OUTER ENVELOPE MEMBRANE PROTEIN 16 (OEP16) OF PEA CHLOROPLASTS

The protein, a cation-selective channel protein, has been overexpressed in *Escherichia coli* .in the form of inclusion bodies, purified and then folded with detergent on a Ni-NTA affinity column. CD spectroscopy studies and ^{15}N-HSQC NMR spectra revealed that the protein is a folded protein composed of α-helices (Ni da et al., 2011).

CELL WALL FIBRONECTIN-LIKE ADHESION PROTEIN

Proteins immunologically related to human fibronectin and showing affinity for gelatin and heparin are found in the cell walls of epicotyls of germinating peas under salt stress at 3-4 times higher concentrations than in unstressed epicotyls. Plant cell wall proteins facilitate better cell anchorage to the cell wall during salt stress or water deficit and are cell adhesion as well as signaling molecules (Pellenc et al., 2004).

ARABINOGALACTANPROTEIN-EXTENSIN (AGPE) GLYCOPROTEINS

The root nodule interface between the leguminous host cell and the microbial symbiont is pivotal for development and differentiation in the symbiotic association between rhizobium and pea and bean plants. Root nodule extensins, referred to as arabinogalactanprotein-extensin (AGPE), are major constituents of the infection thread matrix. In symbiotically defective mutants of pea demonstrating abnormal growth of infection threads, the AGPE epitope is enriched in the extracellular matrix around infected host cells in the central infected tissue of the nodule and also occurs in the lumen of Rhizobium-induced infection threads, implying a mis-targetting of AGPE resulting from defective growth of the infection threads. Mutants in gene sym33 manifest diminished MAC265 labeling. Labeling is undetectable in infection threads and droplets, in contrast to wild-type nodules, indicating a compositional change in the infection thread matrix of sym33 mutants which may correlate with the lack of endocytosis of rhizobia into the legume cytoplasm (Tsyganova et al., 2009).

FERRITIN

Ferritin from pea seed is composed of 26.5-kDa and 28-kDa subunits with remarkable amino acid sequence homology and yet distinct, indicating that the ferritin is encoded by at least two genes. The data indicate that pea seed ferritin has two distinct types of ferroxidase centers found in the 26.5-kDa and 28-kDa subunits, respectively, different from all known ferritins. Spectrophotometric titration and stopped flow data revealed that 48 Fe(II) ions can be bound and oxidized by oxygen at the ferroxidase sites, showing that all ferroxidase sites play a role in fast Fe(II) oxidation. Nevertheless, in contrast to H and L subunits in equine spleen ferritin (HoSF), the 26.5-kDa and 28-kDa subunits do not collaborate in iron turnover into the inner cavity of pea seed ferritin (Li et al., 2009).

DEHYDRIN

An improved method for purification of from soy dehydrin involved acidic extraction of soy whey was followed by chromatography on copper charged Chelating Sepharose Big Beads, intermediate hydrophobic interaction chromatography on Source 15 PHE, and affinity chromatography on blue Sepharose. The procedure can be adopted for pea dehydrin (Herzer et al., 2003).

CONCLUSION

The foregoing account reveals that a host of enzymes with different catalytic activities and nonenzymatic proteins are produced by the pea *Pisum sativum.*

These proteins and enzymes regulate various aspects of metabolism and physiology in the plant. Some of these proteins, like the angiotensin converting enzyme inhibitory peptide, have health promoting actions in human. The pea antifungal proteins, protease inhibitors and lectins may also have antimicrobial and anticancer activities similar to their counterparts from other plants (Chan et al., 2012; Fang et al., 2012; Wong et al., 2010, 2012; Wu et al., 2011). Continued research on *Pisum sativum* will undoubtedly disclose more proteins and enzymes of importance, leading to a better understanding of the biochemistry, physiology and pathology of the the pea and the possible application of these pea proteins and enzymes to our benefit.

REFERENCES

Asif M, Rooney LW, Ali R, Riaz MN. Application and opportunities of pulses in food system: a review. *Crit. Rev. Food Sci. Nutr.,* 2013;53:1168-79.

Bajaj M, Soni G, Singh CK. Interaction of pea (*Pisum sativum* L.) lectins with rhizobial strains. *Microbiol. Res.,* 2001;156:71-4.

Balsera M, Goetze TA, Kovács-Bogdán E, Schürmann P, Wagner R, Buchanan BB, Soll J, Bölter B. Characterization of Tic110, a channel-forming protein at the inner envelope membrane of chloroplasts, unveils a response to Ca(2+) and a stromal regulatory disulfide bridge. *J. Biol. Chem.,* 2009;284:2603-16.

Barranco-Medina S, López-Jaramillo FJ, Bernier-Villamor L, Sevilla F, Lázaro JJ. Cloning, overexpression, purification and preliminary crystallographic studies of a mitochondrial type II peroxiredoxin from *Pisum sativum. Acta. Crystallogr. Sect. F Struct. Biol. Cryst. Commun.,* 2006;62(Pt 7):695-8.

Belenghi B, Salomon M, Levine A. Caspase-like activity in the seedlings of *Pisum sativum* eliminates weaker shoots during early vegetative development by induction of cell death. *J. Exp. Bot.,* 2004;55(398):889-97.

Blöchl A, Peterbauer T, Hofmann J, Richter A. Enzymatic breakdown of raffinose oligosaccharides in pea seeds. *Planta,* 2008;228:99-110.

Bozzo GG, Basset GJ, Naponelli V, Noiriel A, Gregory JF 3rd, Hanson AD. Characterization of the folate salvage enzyme p-aminobenzoylglutamate hydrolase in plants. *Phytochemistry,* 2008 Jan;69:29-37.

Buchner P, Rochat C, Wuillème S, Boutin JP.Characterization of a tissue-specific and developmentally regulated beta-1,3-glucanase gene in pea (*Pisum sativum*). *Plant. Mol. Biol.,* 2002;49(2):171-86.

Castillo J, Zúñiga A, Franco L, Rodrigo MI. A chromatin-associated protein from pea seeds preferentially binds histones H3 and H4. *Eur. J. Biochem.,* 2002 Sep;269(18):4641-8.

Cavada BS, da Silva LI, Ramos MV, Galvani FR, Grangeiro TB, Leite KB, Assreuy AM, Cajazeiras JB, Calvete JJ. Seed lectin from *Pisum arvense*: isolation, biochemical characterization and amino acid sequence. Protein Pept Lett. 2003;10(6):607-17.

Chan YS, Wong JH, Fang EF, Pan W, Ng TB. Isolation of a glucosamine bindingleguminous lectin with mitogenic activity towards splenocytes and anti-proliferative activity towards tumor cells. *PLoS One,* 2012;7(6):e38961.

Del Río LA, Palma JM. Glutathione reductase from pea leaves: response to abiotic stress and characterization of the peroxisomal isozyme. *New Phytol.,* 2006;170:43-52.

Dun XP, Li FF, Wang JH, Chen ZW. The effect of pea albumin 1F on glucose metabolism in mice. *Peptides,* 2008;29:891-7.

Dwevedi A, Kayastha AM. A beta-galactosidase from pea seeds (PsBGAL): purification, stabilization, catalytic energetics, conformational heterogeneity, and its significance. *J. Agric. Food Chem.,* 2009;57:7086-96.

Fang EF, Bah CS, Wong JH, Pan WL, Chan YS, Ye XJ, Ng TB. A potential humanhepatocellular carcinoma inhibitor from Bauhinia purpurea L. seeds: from purification to mechanism exploration. *Arch. Toxicol.,* 2012;86:293-304.

Gucciardo S, Wisniewski JP, Brewin NJ, Bornemann S. A germin-like protein with superoxide dismutase activity in pea nodules with high protein sequence identity to a putative rhicadhesin receptor. *J. Exp. Bot.,* 2007;58:1161-71.

Herzer S, Kinealy K, Asbury R, Beckett P, Eriksson K, Moore P. Purification of native dehydrin from Glycine Max cv., *Pisum sativum,* and

Rosmarinum officinalis by affinity chromatography. *Protein. Expr. Purif.*, 2003;28(2):232-40.

Jager CE, Symons GM, Nomura T, Yamada Y, Smith JJ, Yamaguchi S, Kamiya Y, Weller JL, Yokota T, Reid JB. Characterization of two brassinosteroid C-6 oxidase genes in pea. *Plant Physiol.,* 2007 Apr;143(4):1894-904.

Jakubczyk A, Karaś M, Baraniak B, Pietrzak M. The impact of fermentation and in vitro digestion on formation angiotensin converting enzyme (ACE) inhibitory peptides from pea proteins. *Food Chem.,* 2013;141(4):3774-80.

Jang HK, Lee SW, Lee YH, Hahn TR. Purification and characterization of a recombinant pea cytoplasmic fructose-1,6-bisphosphatase. *Protein Expr. Purif.,* 2003;28(1):42-8.

Jones AL, Gane AM, Herbert D, Willey DL, Rutter AJ, Kille P, Dancer JE, Harwood JL. Beta-ketoacyl-acyl carrier protein synthase III from pea (*Pisum sativum* L.):properties, inhibition by a novel thiolactomycin analogue and isolation of a cDNA clone encoding the enzyme. *Planta,* 2003;216(5):752-61.

Jouvensal L, Quillien L, Ferrasson E, Rahbé Y, Guéguen J, Vovelle F. PA1b, an insecticidal protein extracted from pea seeds (*Pisum sativum*): 1H-2-D NMR study and molecular modeling. *Biochemistry,* 2003;42(41):11915-23.

Kimber MS, Coleman JR, Pai EF. beta-carbonic anhydrase from *Pisum sativum*: crystallization and preliminary X-ray analysis. *Acta Crystallogr. D Biol. Crystallogr.,* 2000; 56(Pt 7):927-9.

Lester DR, Phillips A, Hedden P, Andersson I. Purification and kinetic studies of recombinant gibberellin dioxygenases. *BMC Plant Biol.,* 2005 Sep 25;5:19.

Kim D, Lee G, Chang M, Park J, Chung Y, Lee S, Lee TK. Purification and biochemical characterization of insoluble acid invertase (INAC-INV) from pea seedlings. *J. Agric. Food Chem.,* 2011;59(20):11228-33.

Li C, Hu X, Zhao G. Two different H-type subunits from pea seed (*Pisum sativum*) ferritin that are responsible for fast Fe(II) oxidation. Biochimie. 2009;91(2):230-9.

Meisner AK(, Saffert A, Schreier P, Schön A. Fatty acid alpha-dioxygenase from *Pisum sativum*: temporal and spatial regulation during germination and plant development. *J. Plant Physiol.,* 2009;166(4):333-43.

Ni da Q, Zook J, Klewer DA, Nieman RA, Soll J, Fromme P. Isolation, folding and structural investigations of the amino acid transporter OEP16. *Protein Expr. Purif.,* 2011;80(2):157-68.

O'Kane FE, Happe RP, Vereijken JM, Gruppen H, van Boekel MA. Characterization of pea vicilin. 1. Denoting convicilin as the alpha-subunit of the Pisum vicilin family. *J. Agric. Food Chem.,* 2004;52(10):3141-8.

Pellenc D, Schmitt E, Gallet O. Purification of a plant cell wall fibronectin-like adhesion protein involved in plant response to salt stress. *Protein Expr. Purif.,* 2004;34(2):208-14.

Ortiz-Masia D, Perez-Amador MA, Carbonell P, Aniento F, Carbonell J, Marcote MJ. Characterization of PsMPK2, the first C1 subgroup MAP kinase from pea (*Pisum sativum* L.). *Planta,* 2008;227(6):1333-42.

Ostrowski M, Jakubowska A. Identification of enzyme activity that conjugates indole-3-acetic acid to aspartate in immature seeds of pea (*Pisum sativum*). *J. Plant Physiol.,* 2008;165(5):564-9.

Pandey S, Tiwari SB, Tyagi W, Reddy MK, Upadhyaya KC, Sopory SK. A Ca2+/CaM-dependent kinase from pea is stress regulated and *in vitro* phosphorylates a protein that binds to AtCaM5 promoter. *Eur. J. Biochem.,* 2002; 269(13):3193-204.

Peterbauer T, Mach L, Mucha J, Richter A. Functional expression of a cDNA encoding pea (*Pisum sativum* L.) raffinose synthase, partial purification of the enzyme from maturing seeds, and steady-state kinetic analysis of raffinose synthesis. *Planta,* 2002 Sep;215(5):839-46.

Rahbé Y, Ferrasson E, Rabesona H, Quillien L. Toxicity to the pea aphid Acyrthosiphon pisum of anti-chymotrypsin isoforms and fragments of Bowman-Birk protease inhibitors from pea seeds. *Insect. Biochem. Mol. Biol.,* 2003;33(3):299-306.

Romero-Puertas MC, Corpas FJ, Sandalio LM, Leterrier M, Rodríguez-Serrano M, Meisner AK, Saffert A, Schreier P, Schön A. Fatty acid alpha-dioxygenase from *Pisum sativum*: temporal and spatial regulation during germination and plant development. *J. Plant. Physiol.,* 2009;166(4):333-43.

Sanan-Mishra N, Pham XH, Sopory SK, Tuteja N. Pea DNA helicase 45 overexpression in tobacco confers high salinity tolerance without affecting yield. *Proc. Natl. Acad. Sci. USA,* 2005 J;102(2):509-14.

Scherbak N, Brosché M, Ala-Häivälä A, Strid H, Ohrfelt A, Nilsson F, Strid A. Expression of *Pisum sativum* SAD polypeptides in production hosts and in planta: tetrameric organization of the protein. *Protein Expr. Purif.,* 2009;63(1):18-25.

Shitov AV, Pobeguts OV, Smolova TN, Allakhverdiev SI, Klimov VV. Manganese-dependent carboanhydrase activity of photosystem II proteins. *Biochemistry,* (Mosc). 2009; 74(5):509-17.

Slezack S, Negrel J, Bestel-Corre G, Dumas-Gaudot E, Gianinazzi S. Purification and partial amino acid sequencing of a mycorrhiza-related chitinase isoform from Glomus mosseae-inoculated roots of *Pisum sativum* L. *Planta,* 2001;213 (5):781-7.

Srivastava PK, Singh DS. Isolation and characterization of NADP+-linked isocitrate dehydrogenase of germinating pea seeds (*Pisum sativum*). *Indian J. Biochem. Biophys.,* 2001;38(5):335-41.

Tsyganova AV, Tsyganov VE, Findli KK, Borisov AIu, Tikhonovich NA, Brevin NG. Distribution of legume arabinogalactanprotein-extensin (AGPE) glycoproteins in symbiotically defective pea mutants with abnormal infection threads. *Tsitologiia,* 2009;51(1):53-62.

Tylichová M, Briozzo P, Kopecný D, Ferrero J, Moréra S, Joly N, Snégaroff J,Sebela M. Purification, crystallization and preliminary crystallographic study of a recombinant plant aminoaldehyde dehydrogenase from *Pisum sativum. Acta Crystallogr. Sect. F. Struct. Biol. Cryst. Commun.,* 2008 Feb 1;64(Pt 2):88-90.

Vashisht AA, Pradhan A, Tuteja R, Tuteja N. Cold- and salinity stress-induced bipolar pea DNA helicase 47 is involved inbprotein synthesis and stimulated by phosphorylation with protein kinase C. *Plant J.,* 2005;44(1):76-87.

Venkataraman G, Goswami M, Tuteja N, Reddy MK, Sopory SK. Isolation and characterization of a phospholipase C delta isoform from pea that is regulated by light in a tissue specific manner. *Mol. Genet. Genomics.,* 2003;270(5):378-86.

Wong JH, Ip DC, Ng TB, Chan YS, Fang F, Pan WL. A defensin-like peptide from Phaseolus vulgaris cv. 'King Pole Bean'. *Food Chem.,* 2012;135:408-14.

Wong JH, Ng TB, Cheung RC, Ye XJ, Wang HX, Lam SK, Lin P, Chan YS, Fang EF,Ngai PH, Xia LX, Ye XY, Jiang Y, Liu F. Proteins with antifungal properties and other medicinal applications from plants and mushrooms. *Appl. Microbiol. Biotechnol.,* 2010;87:1221-35.

Wu X, Sun J, Zhang G, Wang H, Ng TB. An antifungal defensin from *Phaseolus vulgaris* cv. 'Cloud Bean'. *Phytomedicine,* 2011;18:104-9.

Ye X, Ng TB. Isolation of lectin and albumin from *Pisum sativum* var. macrocarpon ser. cv.sugar snap. *Int. J. Biochem. Cell Biol.,* 2001;33(1):95-102.

Ye XY, Ng TB. Isolation of pisumin, a novel antifungal protein from legumes of the sugar snap pea *Pisum sativum* var macrocarpon. *Comp. Biochem. Physiol. C Toxicol. Pharmacol.,* 2003 Feb;134(2):235-40.

Ye XY, Wang HX, Ng TB. Sativin: a novel antifungal miraculin-like protein isolated from legumes of the sugar snap *Pisum sativum* var. macrocarpon. *Life Sci.,* 2000 Jul 7;67(7):775-81.

In: *Pisum sativum*
Editor: Shannell Becket

ISBN: 978-1-63463-230-0

Chapter 3

HEALTH PROMOTING EFFECTS OF THE PEA *PISUM SATIVUM*

***Tzi Bun Ng*[1]*, *Charlene Cheuk Wing Ng*[1], *Helen Chan*[2], *Tak Fu Tse*[2] *and Timothy Tam*[2]**

[1]School of Biomedical Sciences, Faculty of Medicine, The Chinese University of Hong Kong, Shatin, New Territories, Hong Kong

[2]Vita Green Health Products Co., Ltd., Hong Kong

ABSTRACT

Evidence has been presented that pea consumption may facilitate prevention of neural tube defects, increase of satiety and reduction of obesity, inhibition of atherosclerosis, prevention of cardiometabolic risk, reduction of head and neck cancer risk, lung cancer risk, colon cancer risk, reduction of fasting serum concentrations of adhesion molecules and inflammatory biomarkers. Pea has anti-oxidant, anti-inflammatory, immunomodulating, and angiotensin converting enzyme inhibitory activities. Trace elements such as selenium are rich in Canadian field peas, Peas may synergize with whole grains in health promoting effects.

Keywords: Pea, *Pisum sativum*, health promoting effects

---

* Corresponding author. School of Biomedical Sciences, Faculty of Medicine, The Chinese University of Hong Kong, Shatin, New Territories, Hong Kong, China. Email: b021770@mailserv.cuhk.edu.hk.

INTRODUCTION

Pulses include peas, chickpeas, beans, and lentils. Pulses contain almost twice the amount of protein compared to cereal grains. In some regions of the world, legume seeds are the only protein supply in the diet. The majority of legumes contain isoflavones, phytosterols, resistant starch, carbohydrates, alkaloids and saponins (Rochfort and Panozzo, 2007), enzyme inhibitors, phytohemagglutinins (lectins), phytoestrogens, galactose oligosaccharides which may exert beneficial probiotic effects in the large intestine, saponins which may exhibit hypocholesterolaemic and anticarcinogenic activities, and phenolic compounds, which may have antioxidant and anticarcinogenic activities. Pulses have hypocholesterolemic and hypotriglyceridemic actions and leguminous fiber has hypoglycemic activity because it contains more amylose than amylopectin (Marles et al., 2013). The health benefits derive mainly from the concentration and properties of starch, protein, fibre, vitamins, minerals and phytochemicals in peas (Dahl et al., 2012). Dietary intake of phytochemicals may provide health benefits and protection against coronary heart disease, diabetes, hypertension and inflammation (Bouchenak and Lamri-Senhadji, 2013). Pulses have a high content of dietary fiber and complex carbohydrates yielding foods with low glycemic index. Pulses have hypocholesterolemic and hypotriglyceridemic actions and leguminous fiber has hypoglycemic activity because it contains more amylose than amylopectin, helping diabetics to maintain appropriate plasma glucose and insulin levels (Trinidad et al., 2010; Marles et al., 2013; Mudryj et al., 2014). Pea protein, when hydrolysed, may yield peptides with angiotensin I-converting enzyme inhibitory and antioxidant activities. The vitamin and mineral contents of peas may prevent selenium or folate deficiency (Dahl et al., 2012)

Pulses can be utilized in processed foods such as bakery products, bread, pasta, tortillas, snack foods, soups, etc. and in frozen dough foods either as added flour or as fillings. Pulses appear to be ideal for inclusion in designing snack foods, baby, and sports foods due to their nutritious and health promoting effects (Asif et al., 2013).Mature hulls (seed coats) contain chlorophylls a and b, trans-lutein and trace amounts of other carotenoids and pheophytin metabolites. Developing hulls contain chlorophylls a and b, β-carotene, lutein, neoxanthin, violaxanthin, and zeaxanthin,. Green-cotyledon varieties of pea possess higher concentrations of lutein than the yellow-cotyledon varieties. The occurrence of flavonoid-related compounds was correlated only with pigmented seed coat genotypes. The carotenoids and chlorophylls in the hulls split from the green and yellow field pea types have dietary potential as a value-added prospect in food supplements (Marles et al., 2013).

The aim of this article is to review the different health promoting effects brought about by consumption of the pea *Pisum sativum*.

CARDIOMETABOLIC RISK PREVENTION AND INHIBITION OF ATHEROSCLEROSIS BY DIETARY INCLUSION OF PEAS

Adams et al. (2006) furnished evidence for the anti-atherosclerotic action of a diet rich in green and yellow vegetables in a LDL receptor -/-, apolipoprotein B transgenic mouse model of atherosclerosis. The mice were allocated randomly into 2 groups of about 50 animals each and provided with the following diets for sixteen weeks: a group receiving a vegetable-free control diet and another group given the same diet but with 30% (w:w) substituted by an equal-parts mixture of freeze-dried peas, green beans, carrots, corn, and broccoli. Aortic atherosclerosis, as assessed by cholesteryl ester content, was lowered by 38% after feeding with the vegetable-rich diet. Plasma levels of total cholesterol were reduced by 12%, VLDL-cholesterol plus ILDL-cholesterol by 32%, and serum amyloid A by 37%, and the body weight fell by 7%. Hence a diet rich in green and yellow vegetables suppresses the development of atherosclerosis resulting in a diminution in the risk of cadiovascular disease (Adams et al., 2006).

Bazzano et al. (2011) performed a meta-analysis of randomized controlled trials to assess how consumption of non-soy legumes affects blood lipids. Studies were retrieved by searching EMBASE (from January 1980 to July 2009), MEDLINE (from January 1966 through July 2009), and the Cochrane Collaboration's Central Register of Controlled Clinical Trials utilizing as medical subject headings and keywords: fabaceae not soybeans not isoflavones and diet or dietary fiber and cholesterol or hypercholesterolemia or triglycerides or cardiovascular diseases. Bibliographies of all retrieved papers were also searched. Out of the 140 relevant reports, the ten randomized clinical trials which were selected compared a non-soy legume diet with a control diet, lasting for at least three weeks, and described alterations in blood lipid levels during intervention and control. Data on study design, participants characteristics, sample size, intervention methods, duration of treatment, and results were independently processed by 2 investigators using a standardized protocol. Data from ten trials representing 268 participants were studied using a random-effects model. Pooled mean net change in total cholesterol level for subjects receiving a legume diet in comparison with control subjects was -11.8 mg/dL (95% confidence interval [CI], -16.1 to -7.5); and mean net change in low-density lipoprotein cholesterol level was -8.0mg/dL (95% CI, -11.4 to -4.6). The data show that a diet rich in legumes other than soy decreases total and LDL-cholesterol (Bazzano et al., 2011).

Results from controlled trials indicate that dietary pulses (peas beans, chickpeas, and lentils) can help rectify dyslipidemia, but heart health guidelines have considered the beneficial evidence as low. Ha et al. (2014) performed a systematic review and meta-analysis of randomized controlled trials to evaluate how consumption of pulses affected established therapeutic lipid targets for decreasing cardiovascular risk including low-density lipoprotein cholesterol, apolipoprotein B and non-high-density lipoprotein cholesterol. Data were pooled by employing a random-effects model. Our findings suggest that dietary pulse intake significantly reduces LDL cholesterol levels. The authors concluded that the data should be confirmed with trials of longer duration and better quality (Ha et al., 2014).

Pea Consumption Increases Satiety and Reduces Obesity

Observational studies demonstrate that pulse consumption lowers the body mass index and the risk of developing obesity. Intake of pulse enhances satiety over 2-4 h, indicating that the effect of pulses on satiety is at least partially mediated by the quantity or composition of the available carbohydrate. Randomized controlled trials demonstrate a beneficial effect of pulses on weight reduction when pulse consumption is combined with energy restriction, but not when there is no energy restriction. There appears to be a beneficial effect of pulses on short-term (three to twelve weeks) satiety and weight loss during intentional energy restriction, but more studies especially those with a longer duration lasting for one year or longer are required, to study the optimal amount of pulses necessary for weight reduction, and include behavioral elements to surmount obstacles to pulse intake (McCrory et al., 2010).

EFFECTS OF GLYCATED PEA PROTEINS ON BACTERIA

Glycation (non-enzymatic glycosylation) changes the structures and activities of proteins. Glycated pea proteins have a reduced susceptibility to enzymatic digestion and can modify the bacterial intestinal ecosystem and influence human health. Non-glycated pea proteins are better energy sources for *E. coli* 360 and *S. aureus*, which suggests that glycation hinders protein utilization by the bacteria mentioned. The inhibitory effect of non-glycated pea proteins on *E. coli* 22, *E. faecium* and *S. saprophyticus* has also been confirmed (Swiatecka et al., 2010).

ANTIFUNGAL ACTION TOWARD *FUSARIUM OXYSPORUM*

The pea produces several antifungal proteins (Ye et al., 2000; Ye and Ng, 2003; Wang and Ng, 2006; Nucci and Anaissie, 2007) which inhibit the growth of *Fusarium spp. such as F.oxysporum and F.solani.*

TRACE ELEMENTS SUCH AS SELENIUM IN CANADIAN FIELD PEAS

Canada is an important pea exporter. An investigation conducted by Canadian Grain Commission on various elements in Canadian peas disclosed that arsenic, cadmium, mercury and lead levels were below the maximum residue levels established by the FAO and WHO in the Codex Alimentarius. The higher selenium level in Canadian peas and their products may benefit regions in the world with the problem of selenium deficiency (Gawalko et al., 2009).

Anti-Oxidant, Anti-Inflammatory and Immunomodulating Properties of an Enzymatic Protein Hydrolysate from Yellow Field Pea Seeds

Enzymatic hydrolyzates of yellow field pea seed protein displayed potent anti-oxidant, anti-inflammatory and anti-bacterial activities. The antioxidant and anti-inflammatory properties were examined in lipopolysaccharide/ interferon-γ-activated RAW 264.7 macrophages. Pea protein hydrolysate suppressed nitric oxide production and secretion of pro-inflammatory cytokines, tumor necrosis factor-α- and interleukin-6. Feeding of pea protein hydrolysate to mice promoted phagocytotic activity of peritoneal macrophages and the intestinal mucosa immune response. The number of IgA+ cells in the small intestine lamina propria, and the number of interferon -γ+, interleukin-4+, and interleukin-10+ cells increased. IL-6 secretion by small intestine epithelial cells (IEC) was enhanced. Pea protein hydrolyzate might have augmented secretion of interleukin-6 in small intestine epithelial cells by stimulating toll-like receptors (TLRs) family, especially TLR2 and TLR4 because both antibodies against TLR2 and antibodies against TLR4 eliminated interleukin-6 secretion induced by pea protein hydrolyzate (Ndiaye et al., 2012).

Legume Consumption Is Inversely Associated with Fasting Serum Concentrations of Adhesion Molecules and Inflammatory Biomarkers

In a cross-sectional study carried out by Esmaillzadeh and Azadbakht (2012), a dietitian administered validated semiquantitative food frequency questionnaires to 486 Tehrani female teachers for estimation of dietary legume consumption calculated by summing up the consumption of peas, lentils, chickpeas, various beans including broad beans, and chickling vetch. Fasting blood samples were collected for determining serum levels of inflammatory biomarkers and adhesion molecules. Subjects found in the highest tertile of legume consumption had lower serum concentrations of soluble vascular cell adhesion molecule-1 soluble intercellular adhesion molecule-1, and E-selectin compared with those in the lowest tertile. A high legume intake was associated with low serum concentrations of high sensitive C reactive protein, tumor necrosis factor-α, and interleukin-6. There was no correlation between legume intake and serum amyloid A concentrations. Legume consumption is inversely associated with serum concentrations of adhesion molecules and inflammatory biomarkers among Iranian women (Esmaillzadeh and Azadbakht, 2012).

Lack of an Effect on Cognitive Impairment

Rahman et al. (2007) investigated the association between dietary factors and cognitive impairment, employing over one thousand subjects with a mean age of 69 years and mean years of education of 10.7 who were participants in the State-wide Survey of Alabama's Elderly (1986-87). Basic demographic information, Mental Status Questionnaire score, and frequency of consumption of peas and dried beans, vegetables, fruits, bread /cereal, milk, cheese, meat (beef, pork, lamb), chicken or turkey, fish, and desserts, were obtained in an inhome interview.Only cheese consumption was found to be inversely related with cognitive impairment in a simple logistic regression analysis, and in a multiple logistic regression analysis, after adjusting for basic socio-demographic factors and for other dietary factors. In the multiple logistic regression analysis, bread or cereal was inversely associated with, and dessert intake positively associated with cognitive impairment. Peas and beans were devoid of an effect (Rahman et al., 2007).

Anticarcinogenic Activity in the Lungs

The effect of vegetables on changes in gene expression in the lungs of female C57Bl/6 mice was investigated using cDNA microarray technology. The mice were fed one of the following diets for a fortnight: a control diet devoid of vegetables (diet 1); a diet containing a vegetable mixture at 100 (diet 2, 10% dose), 200 (diet 3, 20% dose),or 400 (diet 4, 40% dose) g/kg; or a diet with cauliflower at 70 (diet 5, 7% dose); carrots at 73 (diet 6, 7.3% dose); peas at 226 (diet 7, 22.6% dose); or onions at 31 (diet 8, 3.1% dose) g/kg. The vegetable mixture contained all four vegetables. After the mice were killed, the lungs were removed and total RNA was isolated from the lungs for expression analysis of 602 genes involved in pathways of (anti)-carcinogenesis. The results of this study suggest that individual vegetables have a higher potential of modulating genes (5 from the 8 modulated genes) in favor of lung cancer risk prevention, in comparison with the vegetable mixture (2 from the 7 modulated genes); the other gene modulations are expected to enhance lung cancer risk. The pathways involved were miscellaneous and included cell growth, apoptosis, biotransformation, and immune response. Furthermore, carrots were able to modulate most gene expressions, and most of these effects occurred in processes that favored lung cancer risk prevention. The study provides more insight into the genetic mechanisms by which vegetables, in particular carrots, can prevent lung cancer risk (van Breda et al., 2005a).

Anticarcinogenic Activity in the Colonic Mucosa

van Breda et al. (2005b) studied, using cDNA microarray technology, how vegetable consumption affected gene expression in the colon mucosa of female C57Bl/6 mice. Mice were fed one of the following diets: a control diet without vegetables(diet 1); a diet with 100 g/kg (diet2), 200 g/kg (diet3), or 400 g/kg (diet4) of a vegetable mixture; or a diet with 70 g/kg of cauliflower(diet5), 73 g/kg of carrots(diet 6), 226 g/kg of peas(diet7); or 31 g/kg of onions(diet8).

The vegetable mixture used in diets 2 to 4 consisted of the 4 individual vegetables used in diets 5 to 8: cauliflower (30% wet wt), carrots (30% wet wt), peas (30% wet wt), and onions (10% wet wt). To assess changes in gene expression, colonic mucosal cells were collected after sacrifice of the animals. Genes with altered expression were identified which could account for lowered cancer risk at different stages of colorectal cancer development (van Breda et al., 2005b)

Reduction of Head and Neck Cancer Risk

Freedman et al. (2008) performed a study on 490,802 United States participants of the NIH-AARP Diet and Health cohort using Cox proportional hazard models adjusted for potential confounders from 1995/1996-2000. An inverse relationship was found between intake of fruits and vegetables and risk of head and neck cancer. In models mutually adjusted for consumption of fruits and vegetable, a stronger association was observed in the case of vegetables than fruits. When botanical classification was undertaken, those in the highest tertile of leguminosae (peas, dried beans, and string beans), solanaceae (tomatoes and peppers), rosaceae (peach, plums, nectarines, apples, pears and strawberries), and umbelliferae (carrots) had decreased risk of head and neck cancer, but no significant association was detected for nine other botanical groups. Hence consumption of fruits and vegetables is associated with a diminished risk of head and neck cancer (Freedman et al., 2008).

Anti-Proliferative Effect of Bowman-Birk Isoinhibitor from Pea on HT29 Colon Cancer Cells

Bowman-Birk inhibitors (BBI) are stable under acidic conditions of the stomach and resistant to gastric and intestinal proteases. Sufficient quantities arrive at the large intestine in active form to exhibit anti-carcinogenic and anti-inflammatory actions. Recombinant pea BBI (rTI1B) inhibited the proliferation of human colorectal adenocarcinoma HT29 cells *in vitro* (IC50 = 31μM). It inhibited both trypsin and chymotrypsin, with nanomolar Ki values, whereas the related mutant had no effect on the serine proteases and colon cancer cell growth. The growth of non-malignant colonic fibroblast CCD-18Co cells was not affected by either recombinant protein (Clemente et al., 2012).

Pea Lectin Suppresses Growth of Ehrlich Ascites Carcinoma Cells *In Vitro* and *In Vivo* in Mice

The pea produces a lectin (Ye and Ng, 2001; Kabir et al., 2013) which exerts a growth retarding action on Ehrlich ascites carcinoma cells in vitro as well as in mice by triggering apoptosis and G2/M cell cycle arrest (Kabir et al., 2013).

Ribosome Inactivating Proteins from Pea

Two ribosome inactivating proteins which inhibit protein synthesis in the cell-free rabbit reticulocyte lysate system have been isolated from pea (Lam et al., 1998). Ribosome inactivating proteins have a variety of biological activities including anticancer, immunomodulatory and antimicrobial activities (Ng et al., 2010; Fang et al., 2011).

Potential Synergistic Effect of Peas with Whole Grains

Epidemiological evidence reveals that intake of whole grains reduces the risk of chronic disease. Although pulses (dried beans and peas) and whole grains are dissimilar in structural and physicochemical properties, their nutritional and phytochemical components have the potential of complementing and synergizing with each other in health promoting effects such as prevention and management of chronic diseases as suggested by results of observational and intervention trials (Rebello et al., 2014).

Prevention of Neural Tube Defects by Folic Acid in Pea

Folic acid can be employed to curtail the incidence of congenital abnormalities such as neural tube defects. It is recommended that young females intake folic acid-rich food such as peas, other legumes, cruciferous vegetables, spinach, corn, and oranges (Wilson et al., 2003).

Conclusion

Peas are high in fiber, protein, folate, iron, zinc, and magnesium and low in saturated fat and total fat. Increased intake of dry peas and beans which are economical and nutrient-rich foods beneficial to health could elevate the quality of the diet (Mitchell et al., 2009).Long-term studies to ascertain whether consumption of peas and beans can prevent chronic diseases are highly desirable.

REFERENCES

Adams MR, Golden DL, Chen H, Register TC, Gugger ET. A diet rich in green and yellow vegetables inhibits atherosclerosis in mice. *J Nutr.* 2006;136(7):1886-9.

Asif M, Rooney LW, Ali R, Riaz MN. Application and opportunities of pulses in food system: a review. *Crit Rev Food Sci Nutr.* 2013;53(11):1168-79.

Bazzano LA, Thompson AM, Tees MT, Nguyen CH, Winham DM. Non-soy legume consumption lowers cholesterol levels: a meta-analysis of randomized controlled trials. *Nutr Metab Cardiovasc Dis.* 2011;21(2):94-103.

Bouchenak M, Lamri-Senhadji M. Nutritional quality of legumes, and their role in cardiometabolic risk prevention: a review. *J Med Food.* 2013;16(3):185-98.

Clemente A, Carmen Marín-Manzano M, Jiménez E, Carmen Arques M, Domoney C. The anti-proliferative effect of TI1B, a major Bowman-Birk isoinhibitor from pea (*Pisum sativum* L.), on HT29 colon cancer cells is mediated through protease inhibition. *Br J Nutr.* 2012;108 Suppl 1:S135-44.

Dahl WJ, Foster LM, Tyler RT. Review of the health benefits of peas (*Pisum sativum* L.). *Br J Nutr.* 2012;108 Suppl 1:S3-10.

Esmaillzadeh A, Azadbakht L. Legume consumption is inversely associated with serum concentrations of adhesion molecules and inflammatory biomarkers among Iranian women. *J Nutr.* 2012;142(2):334-9.

Fang EF, Ng TB, Shaw PC, Wong RN. Recent progress in medicinal investigations on trichosanthin and other ribosome inactivating proteins from the plant genus Trichosanthes. *Curr Med Chem.* 2011;18(28):4410-7.

Freedman ND, Park Y, Subar AF, Hollenbeck AR, Leitzmann MF, Schatzkin A, Abnet CC. Fruit and vegetable intake and head and neck cancer risk in a large United States prospective cohort study. *Int J Cancer.* 2008;122(10):2330-6.

Gawalko E, Garrett RG, Warkentin T, Wang N, Richter A. Trace elements in Canadian field peas: a grain safety assurance perspective. *Food Addit Contam Part A Chem Anal Control Expo Risk Assess.* 2009;26(7):1002-12.

Ha V, Sievenpiper JL, de Souza RJ, Jayalath VH, Mirrahimi A, Agarwal A, Chiavaroli L, Mejia SB, Sacks FM, Di Buono M, Bernstein AM, Leiter LA, Kris-Etherton PM, Vuksan V, Bazinet RP, Josse RG, Beyene J,

Kendall CW, Jenkins DJ. Effect of dietary pulse intake on established therapeutic lipid targets for cardiovascular risk reduction: a systematic review and meta-analysis of randomized controlled trials. *CMAJ.* 2014;186(8):E252-62.

Kabir SR, Nabi MM, Haque A, Rokon Uz Zaman, Mahmud ZH, Reza MA. Pea lectin inhibits growth of Ehrlich ascites carcinoma cells by inducing apoptosis and G2/M cell cycle arrest in vivo in mice. *Phytomedicine* 2013;20(14):1288-96.

Lam SS, Wang H, Ng TB. Purification and characterization of novel ribosome inactivating proteins, alpha- and beta-pisavins, from seeds of the garden pea *Pisum sativum*. *Biochem Biophys Res Commun*. 1998;253(1):135-42.

Marles MA, Warkentin TD, Bett KE. Genotypic abundance of carotenoids and polyphenolics in the hull of field pea (*Pisum sativum* L.). *J Sci Food Agric.* 2013 ;93(3):463-70.

McCrory MA, Hamaker BR, Lovejoy JC, Eichelsdoerfer PE. Pulse consumption, satiety, and weight management. *Adv Nutr.* 2010;1(1):17-30.

Mitchell DC, Lawrence FR, Hartman TJ, Curran JM. Consumption of dry beans, peas, and lentils could improve diet quality in the US population. *J Am Diet Assoc.* 2009;109(5):909-13.

Mudryj AN, Yu N, Aukema HM. Nutritional and health benefits of pulses. *Appl Physiol Nutr Metab.* 2014 Jun 13:1-8.

Ndiaye F, Vuong T, Duarte J, Aluko RE, Matar C. Anti-oxidant, anti-inflammatory and immunomodulating properties of an enzymatic protein hydrolysate from yellow field pea seeds. *Eur J Nutr.* 2012;51(1):29-37.

Nelson PE, Dignani MC, Anaissie EJ. Taxonomy, biology, and clinical aspects of *Fusarium* species. *Clin Microbiol Rev.* 1994;7(4):479-504.

Nelson PE, Dignani MC, Anaissie EJ. Taxonomy, biology, and clinical aspects of *Fusarium* species. *Clin Microbiol Rev.* 1994;7(4):479-504.

Ng TB, Wong JH, Wang H. Recent progress in research on ribosome inactivating proteins. *Curr Protein Pept Sci.* 2010;11(1):37-53.

Nucci M, Anaissie E. Fusarium infections in immunocompromised patients. *Clin Microbiol Rev.* 2007;20(4):695-704.

Rahman A, Sawyer Baker P, Allman RM, Zamrini E. Dietary factors and cognitive impairment in community-dwelling elderly. *J Nutr Health Aging.* 2007 ;11(1):49-54.

Rebello CJ, Greenway FL, Finley JW. Whole grains and pulses: a comparison of the nutritional and health benefits. *J Agric Food Chem.* 2014;62(29):7029-49.

Rochfort S, Panozzo J. Phytochemicals for health, the role of pulses. *J Agric Food Chem.* 2007;55(20):7981-94.

Swiatecka D, Kostyra H, Swiatecki A. Impact of glycated pea proteins on the activity of free-swimming and immobilised bacteria. *J Sci Food Agric.* 2010;90(11):1837-45.

Trinidad TP, Mallillin AC, Loyola AS, Sagum RS, Encabo RR. The potential health benefits of legumes as a good source of dietary fibre. *Br J Nutr.* 2010 ;103(4):569-74.

van Breda SG, van Agen E, van Sanden S, Burzykowski T, Kienhuis AS, Kleinjans JC, van Delft JH. Vegetables affect the expression of genes involved in anticarcinogenic processes in the colonic mucosa of C57BL/6 female mice. *J Nutr.* 2005b;135(8):1879-88.

van Breda SG, van Agen E, van Sanden S, Burzykowski T, Kleinjans JC, Delft JH. Vegetables affect the expression of genes involved in carcinogenic and anticarcinogenic processes in the lungs of female C57BL/6 mice. *J Nutr.* 2005a;135(11):2546-52.

Wang HX, Ng TB. An antifungal protein from the pea *Pisum sativum* var. arvense poir. *Peptides.* 2006;27(7):1732-7.

Wilson RD, Davies G, Désilets V, Reid GJ, Summers A, Wyatt P, Young D; Genetics Committee and Executive and Council of the Society of Obstetricians and Gynaecologists of Canada. The use of folic acid for the prevention of neural tube defects and other congenital anomalies. *J Obstet Gynaecol Can.* 2003 ;25(11):959-73.

Ye X, Ng TB. Isolation of lectin and albumin from *Pisum sativum* var. macrocarpon ser. cv. sugar snap. *Int J Biochem Cell Biol.* 2001;33(1):95-102.

Ye XY, Ng TB. Isolation of pisumin, a novel antifungal protein from legumes of the sugar snap pea *Pisum sativum* var macrocarpon. *Comp Biochem Physiol C Toxicol Pharmacol.* 2003;134(2):235-40.

Ye XY, Wang HX, Ng TB. Sativin: a novel antifungal miraculin-like protein isolated from legumes of the sugar snap *Pisum sativum* var. macrocarpon. *Life Sci.* 2000;67(7):775-81.

In: *Pisum sativum*
Editor: Shannell Becket

ISBN: 978-1-63463-230-0

Chapter 4

CHARACTERIZATION OF A REACTIVE OXYGEN SPECIES-RESISTANT HIGH YIELDING MUTANT *R3-1* OF *PISUM SATIVUM* CV. 'ALASKA' WITH HIGH TEMPERATURE-RESISTANT PHENOTYPE

***Kohji Hasunuma*[1,•], *Md. Emdadul Haque*[1], *Osamu Miyoshi*[2] and *Yusuke Yoshida*[1]**

[1]Kihara Institute for Biological Research, Yokohama City University, Totsuka-ku, Yokohama, Kanagawa, Japan

[2]Kanagawa Agricultural Technology Center, Vegetable and Crop Science Research Division, Hiratsuka, Kanagawa, Japan

ABSTRACT

A reactive oxygen species (ROS)-resistant *Pisum sativum* cv. 'Alaska' mutant, *R3-1,* has been reported as a double mutant of transit peptide-NDPK2 Ile12Leu and Lys205Glu and pre-sequence-NDPK3 Pro45Ser [Haque et al. (2010) *Planta* 232:367-382]. The yield of young pods was 2.1-fold higher in *R3-1* than that in the wild-type in the field of Kanagawa Agricultural Technology Center. The yield of plant weights in

• E-mail: kohji.hasunuma@gmail.com, Phone: +81-42-795-1430, Fax: +81-42-799-6045.

R3-1 was 2.0-fold higher than those of the wild-type. The *R3-1* showed phenotypes of seedlings standing in the upward direction and the first leaf opening was very fast. In the case of wild-type the seedlings showed clear bending by fook formation. The *R3-1* mutant also showed slow growth in the upward direction, showing low response to negative gravitropism. The *R3-1* mutant showed a high temperature-resistant phenotype compared to that of wild-type, when the seedlings were grown at 35°C under illumination. The phosphorylation of soluble fractions in the wild type and the *R3-1* of leaves of field grown plants showed an increase in the high-molecular weight histidine kinases with molecular masses of 40, 48, 63 and 70 kDa in the mutant, and in the case of membrane fractions 63 and 72 kDa. The increase in the phosphorylation of these high-molecular weight histidine kinases may be the result of the photoresponses partly via the phytochrome, because the phytochrome mediated increase in the phosphorylation of NDPK2 was established. The molecular mechanisms including singlet oxygen and the resulting calcium release to cytosol from vacuole, microsome and plasma membranes were discussed.

Keywords: High temperature resistant, High yielding, Singlet oxygen ($^1O_2$), Super oxide (O_2^-), Phytochrome mediated photoresponse, High and low-molecular weight histidine kinases, Unsaturated fatty acids

INTRODUCTION

Global warming caused by the increase in the concentration of atmospheric CO_2 by the over-usage of fossil fuels such as petroleum, coal and natural gases, and also the over production of cement by heating $CaCO_3$ promoted us a critical research to accelerate fixing atmospheric CO_2 as carbohydrates providing bio-fuels such as bio-ethanol, bio-oil and bio-gases by use of crop plants (Hasunuma et al., 2011).

To increase the rates of photosynthesis by crop plants we must develop methods to create high yielding mutants of crop plants. We have reported the isolation of an ROS-resistant mutant of *Pisum sativum* cv.'Alaska' (Haque et al., 2008; Haque et al., 2010), harboring point mutations in small-histidine kinases of transit peptide-NDPK2 Ile12Leu and Glu205Lys, and leader sequence-NDPK3 Pro45Ser (Haque et al. 2010). Transit peptide-NDPK2 localized in cytosol and on the surface of chloroplast showed a two-fold-increase in the phosphorylation and enzymatic activities by the two point mutations, Ile12Leu in the transit peptide, and Glu205Lys in the C-terminus region of the enzyme. We established that NDPKs in the membrane fraction and soluble fraction were signal transducers of phytochromes (Hamada and Hasunuma 1994; Tanaka et al., 1998; Ogura et al., 1999). The results of signal transduction of phytochrome in various plants are well known to increase in $[Ca^{2+}]$cyt from unknown storage site of Ca^{2+} (Shacklock et al., 1992). The transient increases in Ca^{2+} concentration in the cytosol via the phytochrome has been well established, although no information on the release of Ca^{2+} from Ca^{2+} storage sites was presented.

As a photoreceptor with an open tetrapyrrole as the prosthetic group, phytochrome will function as a photosensitizer and red light energy adsorbed by phytochrome will be transferred to an ambient triplet oxygen ($^3O_2$) emitting singlet oxygen, ($^1O_2$), which will move very fast at a range of 500 μm over the region of neighboring cell (Luksiene 2003; Ayaru et al., 2005; Hasunuma et al., 2012) and may react with unsaturated fatty acids in the vacuolar and microsomal membranes, as well as the plasma membrane. The reaction of the singlet oxygen to the double bond of unsaturated fatty acids, which forms malone-dialdehyde (MDA) in the vacuolar and plasma membranes (Haque et al., 2010), facilitates pore formation, permitting the influx of Ca^{2+} to the cytosol and the release of Ca^{2+} from the vacuole and the microsome to the cytosol, thus increasing the $[Ca^{2+}]$cyt.

We have also established that the singlet oxygen emitted by the phytochrome will be captured by catalases in the cytosol. The catalases in the cytosol formed a protein complex, with NDPK functioning as an inhibitor of NDPK phosphorylation (Fukamatsu et al., 2003; Yoshida et al., 2006; Wang et al., 2007; Haque et al., 2008; Haque et al., 2010). By the acceptance of the singlet oxygen by catalase, catalase binds the singlet oxygen making it negatively charged, and causing some space in the catalase/NDPK protein complex (Fukamatsu et al., 2003; Yoshida et al., 2006; Haque et al., 2010) and facilitating it to accept ATP and allow phosphorylation. NDPK has also been demonstrated to bind NADH (Wang et al., 2007; Haque et al., 2010) and therefore NDPK/NADH will transfer electrons to catalase/singlet oxygen, releasing superoxide ($O_2^{\cdot-}$) (Hasunuma et al., 2011). The resulting superoxide will react with the unsaturated fatty acids of the vacuolar and microsomal membranes and plasma membrane forming MDA (Haque et al., 2010); pores are formed that permit the influx of Ca^{2+} via plasma membrane and the release of Ca^{2+} to the cytosol from calcium storage sites of vacuole and microsome increasing $[Ca^{2+}]$cyt.

The increase in $[Ca^{2+}]$cyt resulted in the increase in the respiration by mitochondria, resulting in the production of a greater amount of ATP and the inevitable production of superoxide (Giorgi et al., 2012). The high respiration caused by the phytochrome, as well as chlorophyll under strong sunlight will reduce the accumulation of energy as carbohydrates, and finaly lead to a reduced crop yield.

In terms of the emission of singlet oxygen via phytochrome and chlorophyll under strong sunlight to a range of 500 μm, we should study the results of photodynamic therapy (PDT). To kill cancer cells, in a tissue, porphyrin derivative and PO_2 were introduced in the tissue, which was illuminated by two laser lights of different wave-lengths to form forces in the cancer tissues (Luksiene, 2003; Ayaru et al., 2005; Hasunuma et al., 2012). The emission of singlet oxygen from the focus was measured by the phosphorescence from the reaction: -Porphyrin derivative + laser lights + triplet oxygen + PO_2 → Porphyrin derivative exited + triplet oxygen + PO_2 →Porphyrin derivative + singlet oxygen + PO_2 → Porphyrin derivative + P_2O_5 (P_4O_{10})+ phosphorescence (Luksiene 2003, Ayaru et al., 2005, Hasunuma et al., 2012).

The diameter of phosphorescence was 1,000 μm, indicating that the singlet oxygen path length was 500 μm, which is well explained by the life-time of the singlet oxygen was within the range of 0.5 – 4 μsec.

The transfer of the energy of laser lights caused not only the excitation of triplet oxygen to singlet oxygen but also confirmed the energy to move very fast with no reaction with ambient materials with path length of around 500 μm. The path length of 500 μm indicated that the energy accepted by phytochrome will cause a 500 μm range of path length for the singlet oxygen, indicating that it will reach to neighboring cells. The finding indicates that function of the phytocrome was to emit singlet oxygen molecules to neighboring cells causing these to react with unsaturated fatty acids of the plasma membrane and the vacuolar and microsomal membranes, thus conferring these membranes to produce pores that are the actual Ca^{2+} channels in the plasma, vacuolar and microsomal membranes.

Phytochromes will function as an emitter of singlet oxygen, permitting it to move at a range of 500 μm (Hasunuma et al., 2012), creating Ca^{2+} channels in the plasma, vacuolar and microsomal membranes, and increasing $[Ca^{2+}]$cyt, which will lead to the activation of mitochondrial ATP production and inevitably, superoxide production. ATP will function to block the influx of Ca^{2+} and also function to sequester $[Ca^{2+}]$cyt to a calcium storage sites, vacuole and microsome (Hasunuma 1998, Giorgi et al., 2012).

Materials and Methods

Preparation of Wild-Type and *R3-1* and *R3-2* Mutants

Wild-type of *P. sativum* cv. 'Alaska' was prepared by self pollinated line of wild type. The induction of ROS-resistant *R3-1* and *R3-2* mutants was as described in Haque et al. (2008), which were obtained after 8-μM PQ treatment of pea seedlings. The *R3-2* was obtained as a branch of *R3-1* and therefore fundamentally the same line.

Morphological Characterization of Seedlings of Wild-Type and the *R3-1* Mutant

Thirty seeds of wild-type and the *R3-1* mutants were sown in vermiculite (1.5 L) moistened with 1L of $2x10^{-3}$ diluted Hyponex. The plastic dishes (33x28x7 cm) were incubated at 8℃, 8-h light (160 μmol m^{-2} s^{-1}), 16-h dark regime for 30 days. (Figure 1a). The seedlings of earlier stages were photographed at 14 days after sowing of seeds (Figure 1b).

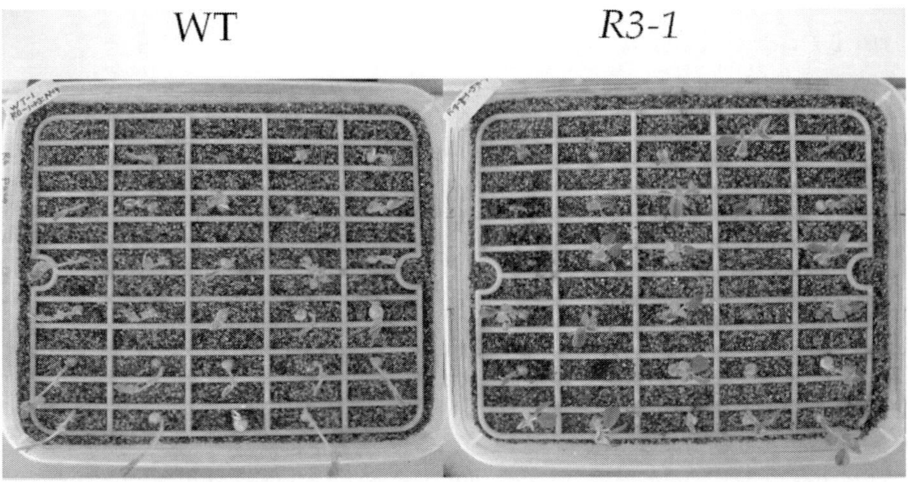

Figure 1a. Early growth pattern of wild-type and the mutant *R3-1*. Seeds of wild-type and the *R3-1* mutant were sown in vermiculite moistened by $2x10^{-3}$ diluted Hyponex under 8-h light (160 μmol m^{-2} s^{-1}) and 16-h dark regime. The cultures were maintained for 30 days.

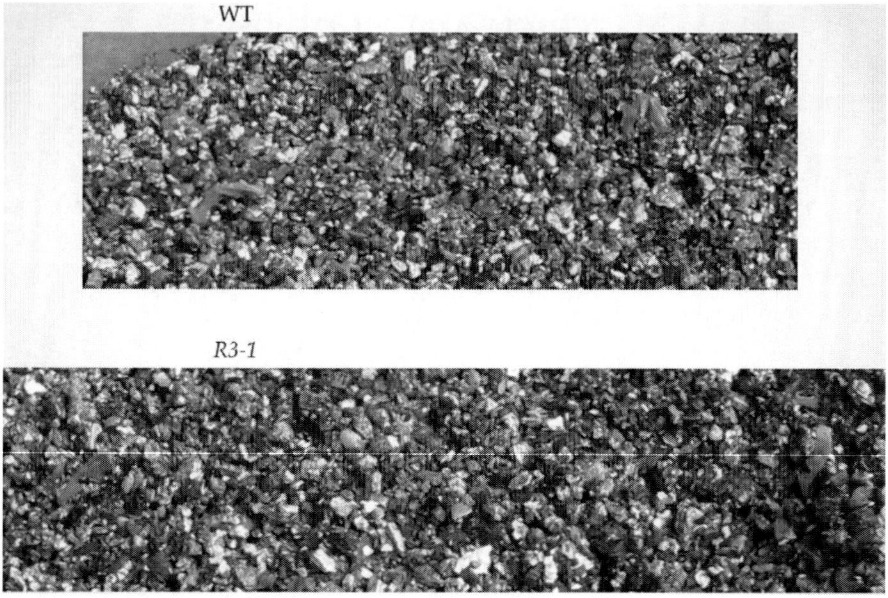

Figure 1b. Growth pattern of very early stage of wild-type and the *R3-1* mutant. The cultures were maintained for 14 days.

Crude Protein Extraction

Leaves from the 1st, 2nd and 3rd position under strong sunlight were harvested at the late vegetative growth stage, covered with foil, frozen in liquid N_2 immediately after harvest, and stored at -80℃. All operations were performed at 0 to 4℃ under infra-red light as a safe-light using a Noctovision system (NVR 2015, Nihon Electric Co., Hamamatsu, Japan), unless otherwise indicated.

Proteins were extracted from the pea leaves by centrifugation, as described by Struglics et al. (1993), with some minor modifications. Leaf residues of wild type and *R3-1* from -80℃ were ground 30 times with a prechilled mortar and pestle into a pea homogenization buffers containing 30 mM Mops (pH 7.3), 3 mM EDTA, 25 mM cystein, and 0.3 M manitol, using 5 volumes of buffer g^{-1} fresh weight, and the homogenates were squeezed through a double layers sheet of nylon cloth. The chloroplasts were sedimented by centrifugation at 4, 000 rpm (4, 000 x g) for 5 min. The resulting supernatant was centrifuged at 10, 000 rpm (10,000 x g) for 10 min to remove cell debris, and the supernatant was centrifuged at 105,000 xg for 30 min. The supernatant to be used as a soluble fraction was aliquated to 0.1 mL and stored at -80 ℃ in the dark. The resulting pellet was resuspended in 2.5 mL of resuspension medium (0.25 M sucrose, 4 mM KNO_3, 5 mM potassium phosphate buffer, pH 7.8, 120 mM N-methyl-D-glucamine, 0.01 mM leupeptine, 0.01 mM pepstatine and 0.5 mM PMSF). The mixture was 10 times homogenized by a small Teflon-glass homogenizer, and 0.1 mL aliquots were frozen at -80 ℃ in the dark. Protein concentration was determined using BSA as a standard, according to the method of Bradford (1976).

Phosphorylation of Proteins by [γ-^{32}P]ATP

The standard reaction mixture (20 μL) contained 4 μL of five-fold concentrated reaction mixture [0.1 M PIPES (pH6.4), 0.5 mM ethylenediaminetetraacetate (EDTA), 0.5 M NaCl, 7.5 mM $MgCl_2$, 1 mM PMSF and 3.6×10^8 Bq [γ-^{32}P]ATP], 2 μL of 1 % triton X-100, 4 μL of resuspension medium containing 0.1 M NaCl, and 10 μL of the soluble faction (5 μg) or the crude membrane (microsomal) fraction. After incubation for 15 sec on ice, the reaction was terminated by adding 12 μL of six-fold concentrated SDS sample buffer containing 10% SDS, 0.125 M TrisHCl, pH 6.8, 2 mM DTT, 10% glycerol and 0.004% bromophenol blue (BPB). The radiolabeled proteins were then fractionated by SDS-PAGE slab gels of 12.5% polyacrylamide essentially as described by Laemmli (1970). The proteins in the gels were transferred to a nitrocellulose filter (pore size, 0.2μm; Schleicher and Schuell, Dassel, Germany) by electroblotting, and the radioactivity on the filter was measured by exposure to a Kodak X-Omat AR film (Boston, MA, USA).

Estimation of Chlorophyll Concentration of Leaf

The relative concentration of chlorophyll in a leaf was measured by SPAD photometer (SPAD-502, Konica Minolta).

Condition of Yield Test Growing Seedlings and Transferring the Seedlings to Field

The yield test of *P. sativum* cv. 'Alaska' was performed in November 2008 using the wild-type (five times self-pollinated) and the mutant *R3-1*. The seeds were provided by Hasunuma, K. Seeds of Narikoma 30 days, and Azumino 30 days as two reference lines were provided by Kanagawa Agricultural Technology Center. On November 27, 2008, seeds were sown in a 72 toray, and the seedlings were transferred to pipe housing for protection against strong wind. The distance between ridges was 120 cm and the distance between plants was 20 cm. For the yield test 10 plants were provided and the trial was repeated twice. To the soil in the field fertilizer N, P_2O_5 and K_2O were provided 1 kg each per 1a. Harvesting of pods from all the plants was performed until May 25, 2009. The plant weights were measured by harvesting a total of 10 plants.

Testing for High Temperature Resistant Phenotype

The 20 surface sterilized pea seeds were imbibed in sterilized deionized water in a sterilized 1-L beaker, and exposed to 35℃ under continuous light (200 μmol m^{-2} s^{-1}) for 7 days and then the seedlings were transplanted to planters. The planters were placed in a glass green house at 23℃ for 30 days and the patterns of growth of wild-type and the *R3-1* mutant were photographed.

RESULTS

The growth Characteristics of Seedlings of the Wild-Type and the Mutant *R3-1*

An early stages of seedlings of the wild-type and *R3-1* indicated that the opening of first leaf was so fast in *R3-1*, compared to that of the wild-type as shown in Figure 1a. In the case of the wild-type very early stages of pea seedlings were characterized by hook formation without opening of the first leaf. We confirmed very early stages of pea seedlings and detected that the wild-type showed bending by hook formation. However, as shown in Figure 1b the mutant *R3-1* germinated stranding upward without hook formation.

Enzymatic Analysis of the Wild-Type and the Mutant *R3-1*

The resistance to strong sunlight will confer the mutant *R3-1* the capacity to produce a high yielding. Under strong sunlight, chlorophyll will be excited to generate triplet chlorophyll, which will result in the excitation of triplet oxygen generated by the photolysis of H_2O to

$$2H_2O \rightarrow {}^3O_2 + 4H^+ + 4e^-$$

to singlet oxygen (${}^1O_2$). Getting energy exciting triplet oxygen to singlet oxygen the process of energy transfer gave much more energy and the singlet oxygen will move at a range of path length of 500 μm.

The soluble fraction and membrane fraction of leaves under strong sunlight from the wild-type and the mutant *R3-1* were prepared as described in Materials and Methods. By use of labeling method of histidine kinase by incubating samples of soluble fraction and the membrane fraction with 10^{-9} M [γ-^{32}P]ATP, high molecular weight histidine kinases, and low molecular weight histidine kinases were labeled. As shown in Figure 2a, we could detect the increase in the phosphorylation of 40, 48, 63, and 70 kDa histidine kinases in *R3-1* in the soluble fraction, and 63 and 72 kDa histidine kinases in membrane fraction compared with those in the wild-type by long exposure of X-ray film.

As shown in Figure 2b obtained by short exposure of X-ray film, the increase in the phosphorylation of these high molecular weight histidine kinases were under the control of low molecular weight histidine kinases of NDPK1 corresponding to 15 kDa, transit peptide NDPK2 corresponding to 19 kDa and leader sequence NDPK3 corresponding to 17 kDa. The increase in the phosphorylation of transit peptide NDPK2 Ile12Leu Glu205Lys mutant molecule of NDPK2 resulted in the faster mobility in the SDS gel electrophoresis, which conferred the enhanced phosphorylation of large molecular weight histidine kinases in soluble fraction and membrane fraction. In our previous study (Haque et al., 2010), we reported that transit peptide NDPK2 Ile12Leu Glu205Lys, the mutant molecule of NDPK2 with glutathione *S*-transferase showed not only enhanced autophosphorylation but also enhanced phosphorelay of the proteins in the soluble fraction (Hasunuma et al., 2012).

Estimation of Chlorophyll Concentrations in the Wild-Type and the Mutants, *R3-1* and *R3-2*

Under strong sunlight, the SPAD values of leaflets from the top of stem (1st leaf), second leaf and third leaf were measured. SPAD values indicate relative concentrations of chlorophyll in the leaflet cells.

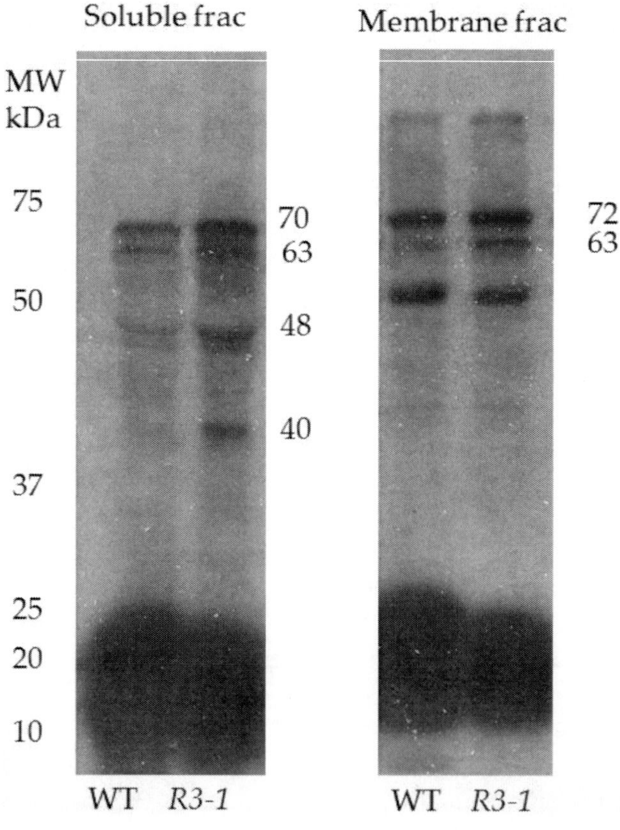

Figure 2a. Proteins in soluble fractions and the membrane fractions of leaves under strong sunlight were labeled for 15 sec by 10^{-9} M [γ-^{32}P]ATP on ice, and the proteins were subjected to SDS-PAGE fractionation. The autoradiography presented was exposed for 3 days.

Five leaflets were measured for the average values ±standard error (SE). As shown in Figure 3, the increases in the chlorophyll concentrations in the mutant leaflets were observed depending on the increase in the number, the first leaflets, the second leaflets, and the third leaflets. The increase in the relative concentrations of chlorophyll in the mutant leaflets may be the result of not only enhanced synthesis of chlorophyll, but also the enhanced protection of chlorophyll degradation against the exposure to singlet oxygen under strong sunlight.

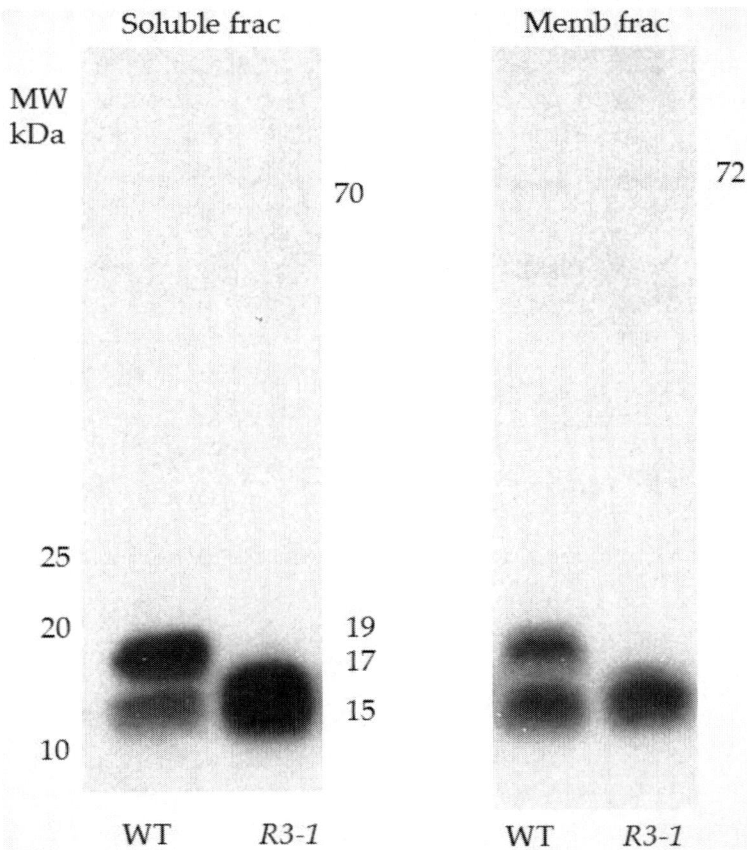

Figure 2b. The same sample as presented in Figure 2a was exposed for 6 h.

The Results of Yield Tests

The following yield tests were performed in Kanagawa Agricultural Technology Center. As shown in Figure 4, the flowering seasons of wild-type and *R3-1* were presented. In the case of the wild-type the plant showed growth upward. However, in *R3-1*, plant showed growth that was not upward, but rather tangled. This pattern of stem growth may reflect the difference in sensitivity to gravity between wild-type and *R3-1*.

The comparison of plant weights dried by blowing air was 2.0-fold higher in *R3-1* compared to that in the wild-type, as shown in Table 1.

The total plants of wild-type and the mutant, *R3-1* with roots were dried in the sunny glass green-house as shown in Figure 5. The plant heights after extension of stems were around 200 cm in both plants. The branching was more frequent in *R3-1* than those in wild-type. The data of Table 2 including Narikoma 30 days and Azumino 30 days as references indicated the date of flower opening in the wild-type was February 13.

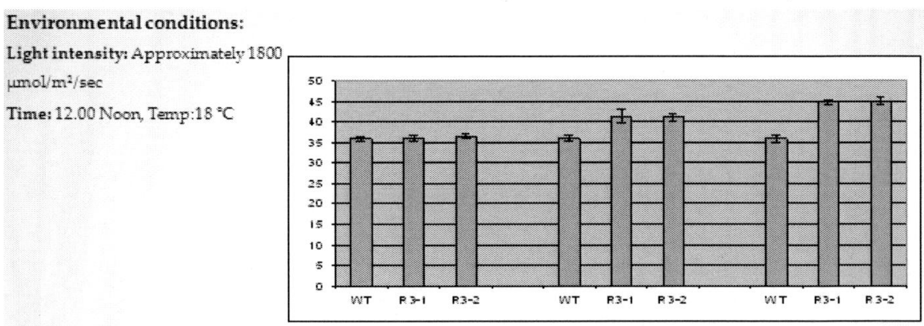

	1st leaf			2nd leaf			3rd leaf		
	WT	R3-1	R3-2	WT	R3-1	R3-2	WT	R3-1	R3-2
Mean	35.82	35.97	36.58	35.98	41.28	41.03	35.97	44.74	44.95
SE	0.62	0.71	0.49	0.76	1.74	1.14	0.93	0.49	0.99
%		0.42	2.12		14.73	14.03		24.38	24.96

Figure 3. The leaves of wild-type and the *R3-1* and *R3-2* mutants under strong sunlight were subjected to measure relative concentrations of chlorophyll by SPAD photometer (SPAD-502, Konica Minolta). Five measurements were performed for the 1st, 2nd, and 3rd leaves and the averages with SE were presented.

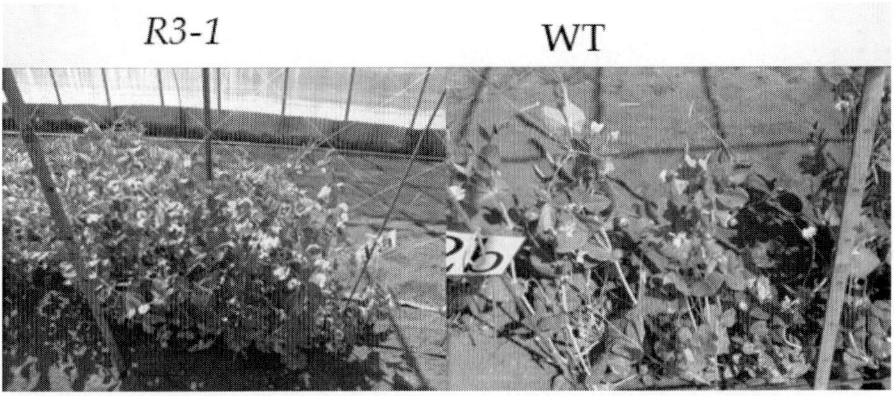

Figure 4. The growing patterns of *R3-1* mutant and the wild-type in the pipe housing of Kanagawa Agriculture Technology Center. The distance of plants was 20 cm and 10 plants were tested. The tests were repeated twice with 2 reference pea plants.

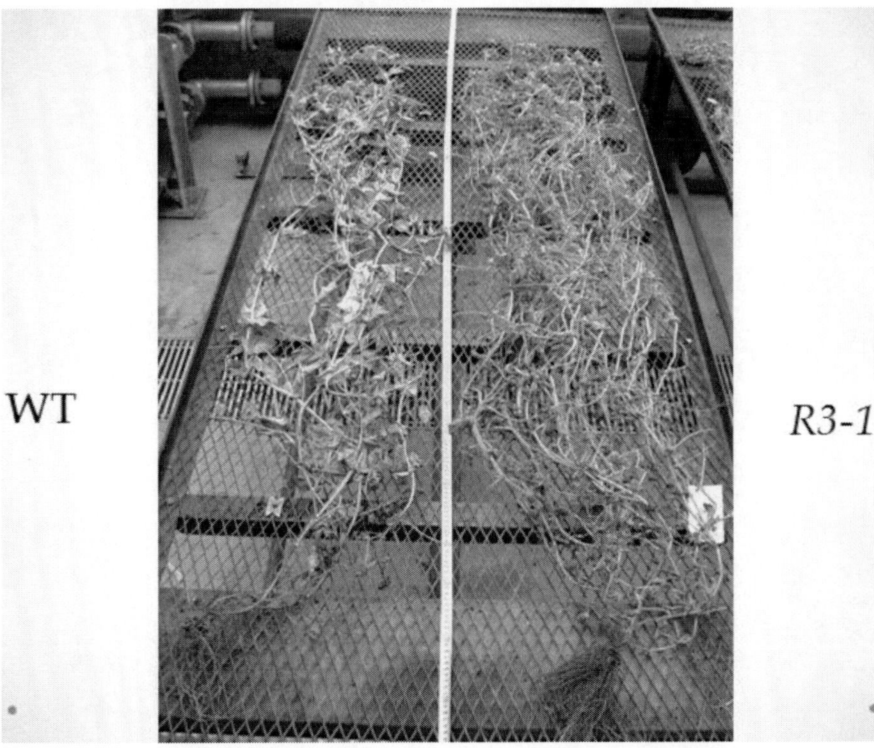

Figure 5. The whole plants of the wild-type and the *R3-1* mutants after removal of pods. Plant heights were around 200 cm.

Table 1.

Weight of total stems and leaves dried by air

	Air dried stems and leaves (g/line)	Dry weight ratio (%)
R3-1	177.7	203.6
WT	87.3	-

Table 2.

	Date of flower opening	Starting date of harvest	Total pod number /line	Pod number *R3-1*/wt (%)	Total pod weight (g/line)	Total pod weight *R3-1*/wt (%)	Average pod Weight (g)
R3-1	20, Mar.	13, Apr.	276	313.6%	439	212.1	1.59
WT	13, Feb.	3, Apr.	88	-	207	-	2.35
Narikoma 30 days	8, Feb.	3, Apr.	224	-	489	-	2.18
Azumino 30 days	8. Feb.	3, Apr.	123	-	301	-	2.45

However, in the case of *R3-1,* the date of flower opening was March 20, and the date of flower opening in *R3-1* was 35 days after the date of flower opening in wild-type. The starting date of pod harvest was April 13 in *R3-1*. However, in wild-type the date of starting of the harvest was 3, April. The total pod number in *R3-1* was three-times larger than that of wild-type. Total pod weight of *R3-1* was more than two-fold higher than that of wild-type. However, average pod weight of *R3-1* was two thirds that in the wild-type.

Eight of representative pods of the wild-type and those of *R3-1* were aligned and we could observe that in the case of *R3-1,* the pods were smaller, as presented in Figure 6.

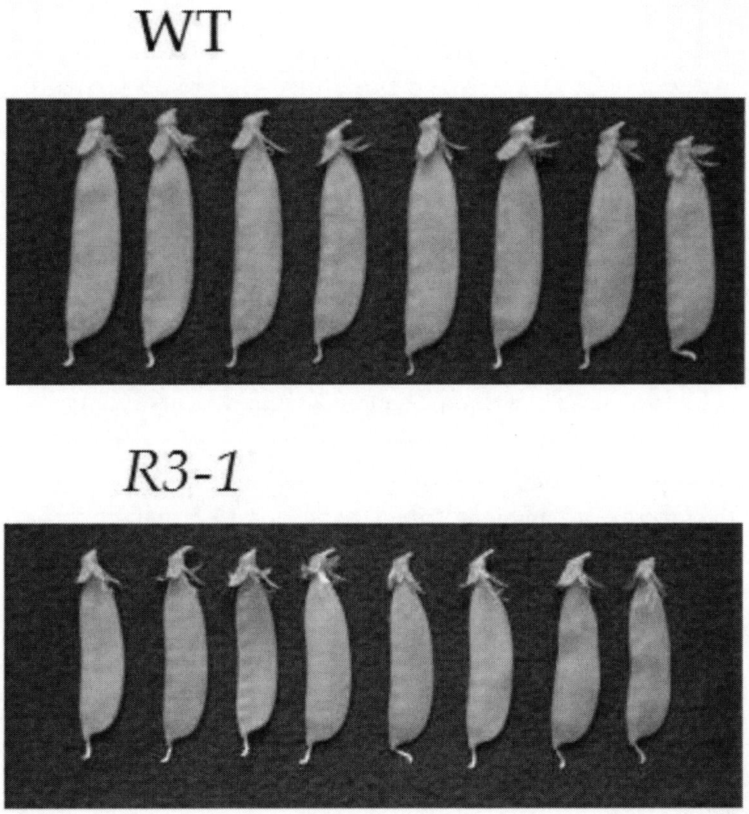

Figure 6. The photograph of pods from the wild-type and the *R3-1* mutants.

The Test of High Temperature Resistance

The test of high temperature resistance was performed by the incubation of imbibing seeds from the wild-type and *R3-1* at 35 °C under light illumination (200 μmol m^{-2} s^{-1}) for one week. The treated germinating seeds were transplanted in 8 planters and 2 seedlings per planter with total of 16 seedlings. We observed that only 4 plants were growing in the case of wild-type. However, in the case of *R3-1*, 10 plants showed good growth. The control experiment testing germination rates of the wild-type and the *R3-1* mutant showed 90% of growth abilities in both lines, as indicated by Figure 1a.

DISCUSSION

Phytochrome mediated responses of pea seedlings were extension of hook and opening of first leaf. In the *R3-1* mutant transit peptide-NDPK2 Ile12Leu Glu205Lys working under the control of phytochrome (Hamada and Hasunuma, 1994; Tanaka et al., 1998; Ogura et al., 1999) showed 2-fold excessive phosphorylation and 2-fold excessive enzyme activity compared to those of the wild-type transit peptide-NDPK2.

These phenomena could well explain the faster extension of hook and faster opening of the first leaf in the *R3-1*. The assumption of the function of phytochrome is that phytochrome had open tetrapyrrole as the prosthetic group, which will function as a photosensitizer (Hasunuma et al., 2012). The acceptance of strong sunlight by phytochrome, as well as chlorophyll will transfer the energy to ambient triplet oxygen ($^3O_2$) and generate singlet oxygen ($^1O_2$), which moves with very fast speed to a length of 500μm. Singlet oxygen will react with unsaturated fatty acids in plasma membrane forming MDA (Haque et al., 2010) and vacuoler and microsomal menbranes generating the channels for Ca^{2+}. As a result, [Ca^{2+}]cyt will increase and mobilize the cytoskeleton to open its hook and open the first leaf in the early stage of seedlings. However, this process will not explain the faster opening of the hook and faster opening of the first leaflet in *R3-1* mutant than those in the wild-type.

Rather catalases in the cytosol form complex with transit peptide-NDPK2 Ile12Leu Glu205Lys in the *R3-1*, and rapidly moving singlet oxygen will be captured by catalases. The capture of singlet oxygen by catalase resulted negatively charged state in the catalase and there appear some space between transit peptide-NDPK2 Ile12Leu Glu205Lys. Because catalase function as an inhibitor of phosphorylation of transit peptide-NDPK2 in the wild-type, the capture of singlet oxygen by catalase will make the inhibiting state to relaxed state conferring the activity to accept ATP for autophosphorylation.

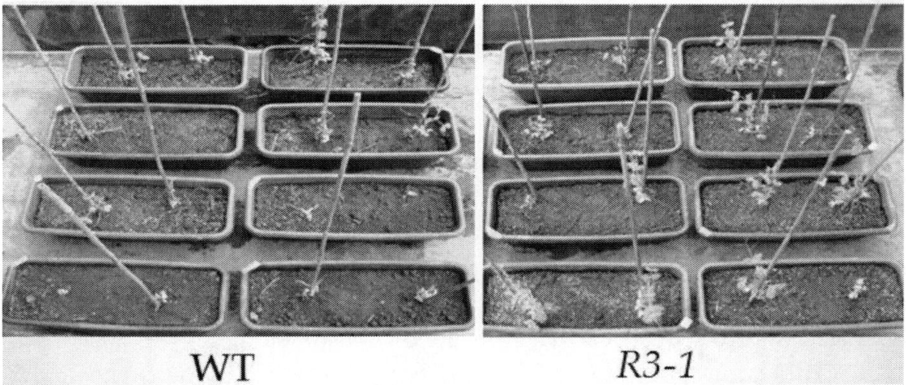

Figure 7. The growth patterns of the wild-type and the *R3-1* mutant in planter after treatment of germinating seeds to expose at 35℃ under light for 7 days.

The mutant molecule of transit peptide-NDPK2 Ile12Leu Glu205Lys will result in faster phosphorylation and subsequent phospho relay to high molecular weight histidine kinases will occur rapidly in the *R3-1*, as shown in Figure 2a. Such a situation will permit the earlier response of hook opening and the faster leaf opening in the *R3-1* mutant than those in the wild-type.

Large amount of transit peptide-NDPK2 in wild-type and transit peptide-NDPK2 Ile12Leu Glu205Lys in the mutant *R3-1* forming complex with catalases in the cytosol will function to supply electron to the singlet oxygen forming a superoxide. The amount of superoxide supplied via the protein complexes will be larger in the *R3-1* mutant, because the rate of autophosphorylation activity of the transit peptide-NDPK2 Ile12Leu Glu205Lys was larger than that in the wild-type. The amount of superoxide supplyed in the cytosol in the *R3-1* will be larger than that in the wild-type, which will easily be detoxified to H_2O_2 and further to H_2O + $^3O_2$ + thermal emission. This situation will confer the *R3-1* mutant to show 2-fold increase in the yield of pods and total plant weights compared with wild-type did.

High temperature resistant phenotype of the *R3-1* mutant will be the result of high activity of transit peptide-NDPK2 Ile12Leu Glu205Lys in the *R3-1*. In *Saccharum officinarum* heat shock of the cultured cells showed enhanced phosphorylation of NDPK (Moisyadi et al., 1994). Further enhanced phosphorylation of the transit peptide-NDPK2 Ile12Leu Glu205Lys in the *R3-1* will phosphorylate high molecular weight histidine kinases by phospho relay (Hasunuma et al., 2012). The function of these high molecular weight histidine kinases was not yet known. However, most of stress responses showed relation to high molecular weight histidine kinases, which will be estimated to have a function of detoxifying ROS, including singlet oxygen. We know that drought resistance was reported to be controlled by histidine kinase (Nongpiur et al., 2012; Xoconostle-Cazares et al., 2011). Histidine kinase activities showed circadian rhythm in cyanobacteria (Iwasaki et al., 2000) and rates of photosynthesis showed circadian rhythm (Hennessey and Field, 1991), which are greatly affected by ROS including singlet oxygen.

We demonstrated that the major component of circadian rhythm was ROS, including singlet oxygen by use of *Neurospora crassa* (Yoshida et al., 2008; Yoshida et al., 2011). Small histidine kinases, NDPK1, (transit peptide-)NDPK2 and (pre-sequence-)NDPK3 were demonstrated directly to concern to the detoxification processes of singlet oxygen and H_2O_2 in *Arabidopsis thaliana, N. crassa* and *P. sativum* cv. 'Alaska' (Fukamatsu et al., 2003; Yoshida et al., 2006; Wang et al., 2007; Haque et al., 2010). The *R3-1* mutant showed retardation of flower bud formation of 35 days, and also showed 2-fold higher phosphorylation and enzymatic activities in small histidine kinase of transit peptide-NDPK2 Ile12Leu Lys205Glu than those of the wild-type. These high activities of phosphorylation of transit peptide-NDPK2 Ile12Leu Lys205Glu will result in the retardation of effective concentration of ROS, including sinlet oxygen, conferring the change of condition to initiate flower bud formation.

The *R3-1* mutant showed a high temperature-resistant phenotype. At high temperatures such as 35°C the rate of respiration will increase. In the case of wild-type, the increase in temperature under light will cause rising up of singlet oxygen emission and increase in pore formation in plasma membrane and vacuolar and microsomal membranes at the unsaturated fatty acids permitting the rising up of $[Ca^{2+}]$cyt. The condition will result in a higher respiration in mitochondria and results in the death of seedlings. However, in the case of the *R3-1* mutant, a high activity of transit peptide-NDPK2 Ile12Leu Lys205Glu, which functions in the detoxyfication of singlet oxygen, will contribute to the reduction in the reactions with unsaturated fatty acids in the membranes triggered by the singlet oxygen (Haque et al., 2010), thus, maintaining higher survival rates at high temperatures than that of the wild-type.

ACKNOWLEDGMENT

We are grateful to Winslow R. Briggs for his continuous encouragement throughout this study. We thank Nissan Motor, Co., Ltd. for assisting in the study, and for providing financial support. This study was also supported by Mishima Kaiun Memorial Foundation, Yamada Science Foundation, and financially by YCU.

REFERENCES

Ayaru L., Bown S. G. and Pereira S. P. (2005) Photodynamic therapy for pancreatic and biliary tract carcinoma. *Intern. J. Gastrointestinal Cancer*, 35: 1-13.

Bradford M. M. (1976) Rapid and sensitive method for the quantification of microgram quantities of protein utilizing the principle of protein-dye binding. *Anal. Biochem.*, 72: 248-254.

Fukamatsu Y., Yabe N. and Hasunuma K. (2003) *Arabidopsis* NDK-1 is a component of ROS signaling by interacting with three catalases. *Plant Cell Physiol.*, 44: 982-989.

Giorgi C., Agnoletto C., Bononi A., Bonora M., Marchi E. D., Marchi S., Missiroli S., Patergnani S., Poletti F., Rimessi A., Suski J. M., Wieckowski M. R. and Pinton P. (2012) Mitochondrial calcium homeostasis as potential target for mitochondrial decline. *Mitochondrion*, 12: 77-85.

Hamada T. and Hasunuma K. (1994) Phytochrome mediated light signal transmission to the phosphorylation of proteins in the plasma membrane and the soluble fraction of etiolated pea stem sections. *J. Photochem. Photobiol. B: Biol.*, 24: 163-167.

Haque Md. E., Yoshida Y. and Hasunuma K. (2008) Paraquat-resistant mutant lines in *Pisum sativum* cv. Alaska: biochemical and phenotypic characterization. *Plant Biotech. Rep.,* 2: 21-31.

Haque Md. E., Yoshida Y. and Hasunuma K. (2010) ROS play an important role in the plant growth and production in ROS-resistant *Pisum sativum* cv. *Alaska. Planta*, 232: 367-382.

Hasunuma K. (1998) Molecular aspects of light signal transduction, circadian rhythm and flowering in plants. *Recent Res. Devel. in Photochem. Photobiol.*, 2: 47-52.

Hasunuma K., Yoshida Y. and Haque Md. E. (2012) Molecular basis of signal transduction of high intensity light via nucleoside diphosphate kinase (NDPK) in *Neurospora crassa* and *Pisum sativum* cv. Alaska. Photoreceptors: Physiology, Types and Abnormalities, Eds Akutagawa E. and Ozaki K. *Nova Science Publishers*, Inc NY pp 149-162.

Hasunuma K., Yoshida Y., Haque Md. E., Wang N., Fukamatsu Y., Miyoshi O. and Lee B. (2011) Global warming, plant paraquat resistance, and light signal transduction through nucleoside diphosphate kinase as a paradigm for increasing food supply. *Naunyn-Schmidberg's Arch. Pharmacol.,* 384 (4-5): 391-395.

Hennessey T. L. and Field C. B. (1991) Circadian rhythms in photosynthesis oscillations in carbon assimilation and stomatal conductance under constant conditions. *Plant Physiol.,* 96: 831-836.

Iigusa H., Yoshida Y. and Hasunuma K. (2005) Oxygen and hydrogen peroxide enhance light–induced carotenoid synthesis in *Neurospora crassa. FEBS Lett.,* 579: 4012-4016.

Iwasaki H., Williams S. B., Kitayama Y., Ishiura M., Golde S. S. and Kondo T. (2000) A KaiC-interacting sensory histidine kinase, SasA, necessary to sustain robust circadian oscillation in cyanobacteria. *Cell*, 101: 223-233.

Laemmli U. K. (1970) Cleavage of structural proteins during the assembly of the head of bacteriophage T4. *Nature,* 227: 680.

Lee S., Vu D. H., Hinds M. F., Davis S. J., Liang A. and Hasan T. (2008) Pulsed diode laser-based singlet oxygen monitor for photodynamic therapy: in vivo studies of tumor-laden rats. *J. Biomed. Opt.*, 13(6): 064035.

Luksiene Z. (2003) Photodynamic therapy: mechanism of action and ways to improve the efficiency of treatment. *Medicina,* 39: 1137-1150.

Moisyadi S., Dharmasiri S., Harrington H. M. and Lukas T. J. (1994) Characterization of a low molecular mass autophosphorylating protein in cultured sugarcane cells and its identification as a nucleoside diphosphate kinase. *Plant Physiol.,* 104: 1401-1409.

Nongpiur R., Soni P., Karan R., Singla-Pareek S. L. and Pareek A. (2012) Histidine kinases in plants – cross talk between hormone and stress responses – *Plant Signal Behave*, 7: 1230-1237.

Ogura T., Tanaka N., Yabe N., Komatsu S. and Hasunuma K. (1999) Characterization of protein complexes containing NDP kinase with characteristics of light signal transduction through phytochrome in etiolated pea seedlings. *Photochem. Photobiol.*, 69: 397-403.

Shacklock P. S., Read N. D. and Trewavas A. J. (1992) Cytosolic free calcium mediates red light-induced photomorphogenesis. *Nature*, 358: 753-755.

Struglics A., Fredlund K. M., Rasmusson A. G. and Moller I. M. (1993) The presence of a short redox chain in the membrane of intact potato tuber peroxisomes and the association of malate dehydrogenase with the peroxisomal membrane. *Physiologia Plantarum*, 88: 19-28.

Tanaka N., Ogura T., Noguchi T., Hirano H., Yabe N. and Hasunuma K. (1998) Phytochrome-mediated light signals are transduced to nucleoside diphosphate kinase in *Pisum sativum* L cv. Alaska. *J. Photochem. Photobiol. B:Biol.,* 45: 113-121.

Treverg J. R., Quinlan C. L. and Brand M. D. (2011) Evidence for two sites of superoxide production by mitochondrial NADH-ubiquinone oxidoreductase (complex I). *J. Biol. Chem.,* 286: 27103-27110.

Wang N., Yoshida Y. and Hasunuma K. (2007) Catalase-1 (CAT-1) and nucleoside diphosphate kinase-1 (NDK-1) play an important role in protecting conidial viability under light stress in *Neurospora crassa. Mol. Genet. Genomics*, 278: 235-242.

Xoconostle-Cazares B., Ramirez-Ortega F. A., Flores-Elenes L. and Ruiz-Medrano R. (2011) Drought tolerance in crop plants. *Am. J. Plant Phys.*, 5: 1-16.

Yoshida Y., Maeda T., Lee B. and Hasunuma K. (2008) Conidiation rhythm and light entrainment in superoxide dismutase mutant in *Neurospora crassa. Mol. Genet. Genomics,* 279: 193-202.

Yoshida Y., Iigusa H., Wang N. and Hasunuma K. (2011) Cross-talk between the cellular redox state and circadian system in Neurospora. *PloS ONE,* 6(11): e28227: 1-11.

Yoshida Y., Ogura Y. and Hasunuma K. (2006) Interaction of nucleoside diphosphate kinase and catalases for stress and light responses in *Neurospora crassa. FEBS Lett.*, 580: 3282-3286.

In: *Pisum sativum*
Editor: Shannell Becket
ISBN: 978-1-63463-230-0

Chapter 5

NUTRITION-STRUCTURE INTERACTIONS IN GREEN-TYPE AND YELLOW-TYPE PEAS (*PISUM SATIVUM*): MOLECULAR FUNCTIONAL GROUPS MAINLY RELATED TO LIPID BIOPOLYMER

***Gloria Q. Yu*[1,2], *Zhiyuan Niu*[1] *and Peiqiang Yu*[1,*]**
[1]Department of Animal and Poultry Science, College of Agriculture and Bioresources, the University of Saskatchewan, Saskatoon, SK, Canada
[2]Advanced IRP Program, Walter Murray Collegiate, Saskatoon, Canada

ABSTRACT

To date, there is limited study on structural profiles on a molecular level mainly related to lipid biopolymers in different type of peas. This research aims to determine molecular structural features of lipid that mainly related to functional groups in the recently developed Green-type and Yellow-type CDC pea varieties: CDC Strike (Green-Type) vs. CDC Meadow (Yellow-Type) and relatively quantify the antisymmetric CH3 ("CH_3as") and CH2 ("CH_2as") (ca. 2960 and 2923 cm (-1), respectively), symmetric CH3 ("CH_3s") and CH2 ("CH_2s") (ca. 2873 and 2954 cm (-1),

[*] Corresponding author contact: Dr. Peiqiang Yu, Professor and Ministry of Agriculture Strategic Research Chair, University of Saskatchewan, Canada; Tel: (306) 966 4132, E-mail: peiqiang.yu@usask.ca.

respectively) functional groups and carbonyl C=O ester (ca. 1745 cm (-1) spectral intensities as well as their ratios of antisymmetric CH(3) to antisymmetric CH(2) (Ratio of CH_3as to CH_2as), ratios of symmetric CH(3) to symmetric CH(2) (Ratio of CH_3s to CH_2s), and ratios of carbonyl C=O ester peak area to total CH peak area (Ratio of C=O ester to CH). Together with the multivariate molecular spectral analyses, the study focused on detecting spectral feature of molecular structure functional groups that are related to lipid biopolymer in different types of peas.

Keywords: Nutrition-structure interactions, yellow and green types of peas, cultivation, functional groups, lipid conformation, structural modification and spectral features

1. INTRODUCTION

Two types of green-type and yellow-type of peas (*Pisum sativum)* varieties have been developed by Crop Development Center (CDC, the University of Saskatchewan, Saskatoon), such as Green-Type: cv. CDC Strike and Yellow-Type: cv. CDC Meadow (Warkentin et al., 2007; The Western Producer, 2014).

To date, there is limited study on structural profiles on a molecular level mainly related to lipid biopolymers in different type of peas. This research aims to determine molecular structural features of lipid that mainly related to functional groups in the recently developed Green-type and Yellow-type CDC pea varieties: CDC Strike (Green-Type) vs. CDC Meadow (Yellow-Type) and relatively quantify the antisymmetric CH3 ("CH_3as") and CH2 ("CH_2as") (ca. 2960 and 2923 cm (-1), respectively), symmetric CH3 ("CH_3s") and CH2 ("CH_2s") (ca. 2873 and 2954 cm (-1), respectively) functional groups and carbonyl C=O ester (ca. 1745 cm (-1) spectral intensities as well as their ratios of antisymmetric CH(3) to antisymmetric CH(2) (Ratio of CH_3as to CH_2as), ratios of symmetric CH(3) to symmetric CH(2) (Ratio of CH_3s to CH_2s), and ratios of carbonyl C=O ester peak area to total CH peak area (Ratio of C=O ester to CH).

The multivariate molecular spectral analyses, cluster analysis and principal component analysis of original spectra (without spectral parameterization), distinguished the structural differences in the antisymmetric and symmetric CH(3) and CH(2) spectral region (ca. 3001-2799 cm(-1)) and carbonyly C=O ester band region (ca. 1771-1714 cm(-1)). The emphasis of this study focused on how molecular structure functional groups that are related to lipid biopolymer could be detected using molecular spectroscopic techniques with multivariate techniques.

2. Lipid Related Molecular Structural Spectral Features of Green Type and Yellow-Type of CDC Peas (*Pisum sativum*): Comparison Between Different Tpes

The molecular structures can be detected by advanced molecular spectroscopy such as FT/IR-ATR molecular spectroscopy (Yu, 2010; Samadi and Yu, 2011). In this project, we aimed to use univeriate molecular spectral analysis method to determine molecular structural changes of lipid related functional groups in the Green-type and Yellow-type CDC pea varieties.

2.1. Green-Type and Yellow-Type of CDC Peas (*Pisum sativum*)

The Green-type and Yellow-type CDC pea varieties: CDC Strike (Green-Type) vs. CDC Meadow (Yellow-Type), were provided by Professor Dr. Tom Warkentin, Crop Development Centre (CDC, University of Saskatchewan, Saskatoon, Canada).

2.2. Green-Type and Yellow-Type of CDC Peas (*Pisum sativum*): Univariate Approach

Molecular functional groups that are related to lipid biopolymer in the green-type and yellow-type of CDC peas (*Pisum sativum*) were identified according to published reports (Himmelsbach et al., 1998; Wetzel et al., 1998; Marinkovic and Chance, 2006; Yu, 2011) and analyzed using univariate molecular spectral analysis (Yu, 2004). Figure 1 shows typical spectrum in green-type (CDC Strike) of peas.

Functional groups that are related to lipid biopolymers included antisymmetric CH_3 (at ca. 2960 cm^{-1}), antisymmetric CH_2 (at ca. 2923 cm^{-1}), symmetric CH_3 (at ca. 2873 cm^{-1}) and symmetric CH_2 (at ca. 2853 cm^{-1}), and lipid carbonyl C=O ester group (at ca. 1745 cm^{-1}). The carbonyl C=O ester group and antisymmetric and symmetric CH_2 and CH_3 stretching functional group band in a typical spectrum in the green-type and yellow-type of CDC peas (*Pisum sativum*) normally located in the region of ca. 1771-1714 cm^{-1} (Figure 2a) and 3001 – 2799 cm^{-1}, respectively.

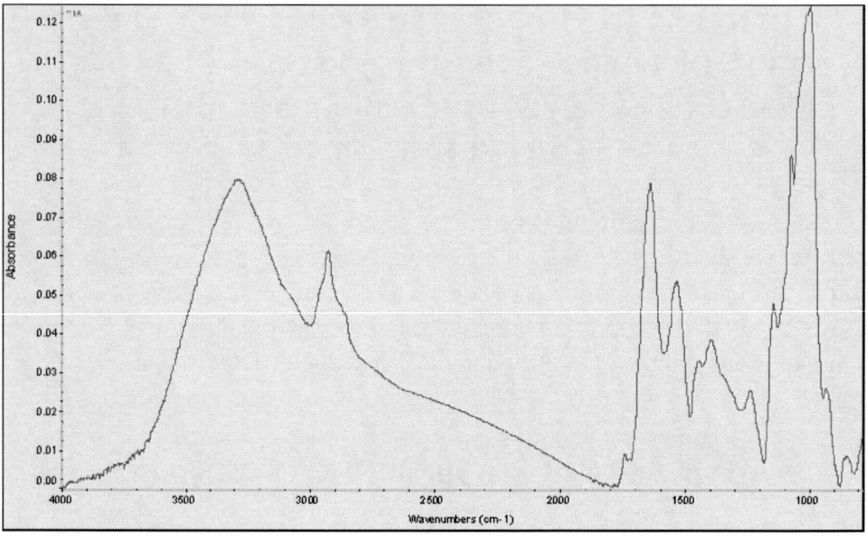

Figure 1. Typical spectrum in green-type (CDC Strike) of peas: 4000-800 cm-1.

The component peaks and frequencies that comprise the antisymmetric and symmetric CH_2 and CH_3 stretching bands in the CH region were identified using the second derivative function. The spectral intensities of peak height and area of the component bands representing antisymmetric CH_2 and CH_3 stretching functional group bands and their ratios in the original spectra were calculated (Figures 2b). Statistical analyses of spectral intensity of height, area and ratios of different molecular functional groups (antisymmetric CH_3 and antisymmetric CH_2 functional groups, symmetric CH_3 and symmetric CH_2 functional groups, as well as carbonyl C=O ester group) were performed using the MIXED procedure of SAS (version 9.1.3). The contrast statement was used to compare between the raw and the heated seed samples. For all statistical analyses, significance was declared at $P < 0.05$. Differences among the treatments were evaluated using a multiple comparison test following the Tukey method.

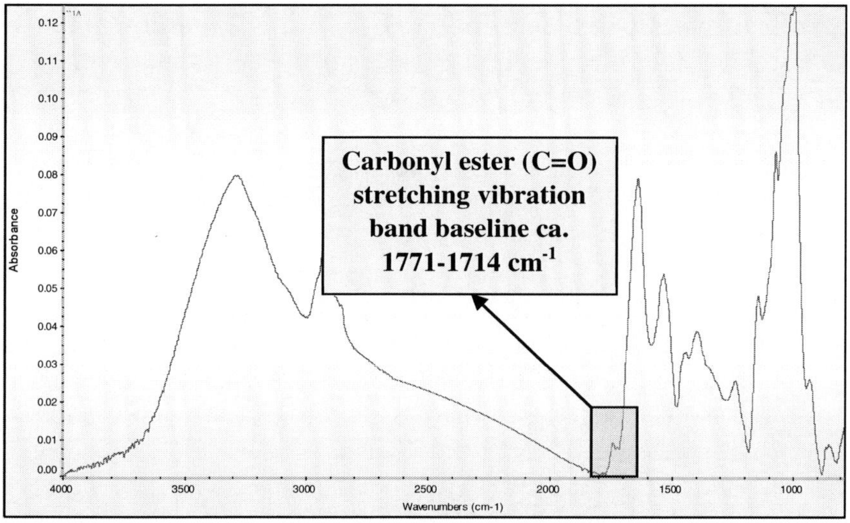

(a) Typical spectral bands that mainly associate with lipid in peas.

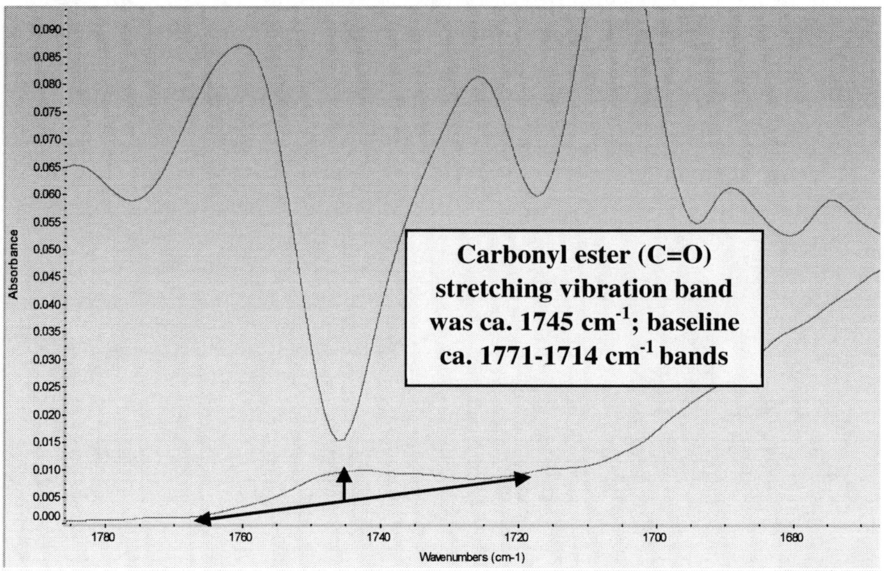

(b) Carbonyl ester (C=O) stretching vibration band ca. 1745 cm^{-1}; baseline ca. 1767-1710 cm.[1]

Figure 2. Typical FTIR-ATR spectrum in CDC peas in the mid-IR region ca. 4000-800 cm-1 (a) showing function groups that mainly associated with lipid: (b). carbonyl ester (C=O) stretching vibration band was ca. 1745 cm-1; baseline ca. 1771-1714 cm-1.

2.3. Antisymmetric and Symmetric CH_3 and CH_2 and Carbonyl C=O Ester Molecular Spectral Profiles of Green-Type and Yellow-Type of CDC Peas (*Pisum sativum*)

Tables 1-3 shows molecular structure spectral features of CH functional groups in terms of the peak height of CH3-antisymmetric (CH3as), CH2-antisymmetric (CH2as), CH3-symmetric (CH3s), CH2-symmetric (CH2s), carbonyl C=O ester and their ratios of yellow type and green type of CDC peas. The results indicated there were no significant differences between the green-type (cv. CDC Strike) and yellow-type (cv. CDC Meadow) of CDC peas in spectral peak height of CH_3-antisymmetric (CH_3as), CH_2-antisymmetric (CH_2as), the ratio CH_3-antisymmetric (CH_3as) to CH_2-antisymmetric (CH_2as) (Table 1) and spectral peak height of CH_3-symmetric (CH_3s), CH_2-symmetric (CH_2s), the ratio CH_3-symmetric (CH_3s) to CH_2-symmetric (CH_2s) (Table 2), but significant differences in both spectral peak height and area intensity of carbonyl C=O ester at 1745 cm^{-1} (Table 3). The CDC Strike (green-type) had higher peak intensity in carbonyl C=O ester, indicating structure conformation at 1745 cm-1 differes (Table 3). There were no significant difference in the ratio of carbonyl C=O ester peak area to total CH (CH3 and CH2) peak area.

Table 1. Molecular structure spectral features of CH functional groups in terms of the peak height of CH_3-antisymmetric (CH_3as), CH_2-antisymmetric (CH_2as) and their ratios of yellow type and green type of CDC peas

Item	Peas Type		
	Green-Type CDC Strike	Yellow-type CDC Meadow	SEM[1]
Peak height of CH_3-antisymmetric (CH_3as) and CH_2-antisymmetric (CH_2as)[2]			
CH_3as	0.0093	0.0089	0.00037
CH_2as	0.0194	0.0181	0.00068
Ratio CH_3-antisymmetric (CH_3as) to CH_2-antisymmetric (CH_2as)			
Ratio of CH_3as to CH_2as	0.4849	0.4909	0.00603

[1]SEM = pooled standard error of means; Means with the different letter within the same row are significantly different ($P < 0.05$).

[2]Peak centers for the CH_3-antisymmetric, CH_2-antisymmetric were ca. 2957 cm^{-1}, 2926 cm^{-1}, respectively and baseline ca. 3021-2800 cm^{-1} for the all CH groups.

Table 2. Molecular structure spectral features of CH functional groups in terms of the peak height of CH_3-symmetric (CH_3s), CH_2-symmetric (CH_2s) and their ratios of yellow type and green type of CDC peas

Item	Peas Type		
	Green-Type CDC Strike	Yellow-type CDC Meadow	SEM[1]
Peak height of CH_3-symmetric (CH_3s) and CH_2-symmetric (CH_2s) [2]			
CH_3s	0.0085	0.0079	0.00028
CH_2s	0.0081	0.0077	0.00028
Ratio CH_3-symmetric (CH_3s) to CH_2-symmetric (CH_2s)			
Ratio of CH_3s to CH_2s	1.0621	1.0348	1.1434

[1] SEM = pooled standard error of means; Means with the different letter within the same row are significantly different ($P < 0.05$).

[2] Peak center for the CH_3-symmetric, CH_2-symmetric groups was ca. 2871 cm^{-1}, and 2855 cm^{-1}, respectively and baseline ca. 3021-2800 cm^{-1} for the all CH groups.

Table 3. Molecular structure spectral feature of carbonyl C=O ester (C=O) in terms of peak height and area and total CH peak area as well as their ratios

Item	Peas Type		
	Green-Type CDC Strike	Yellow-type CDC Meadow	SEM[1]
Carbonyl C=O ester at 1745 cm^{-1} [2]			
Peak height intensity	0.0053 a	0.0042 b	0.00021
Peak area intensity	0.1443 a	0.0858 b	0.00795
Total CH area			
Peak area intensity	1.5066	1.4123	0.05249
Ratio of Carbonyl C=O ester area to total CH (CH3 and CH2) area			
Ratio of C=O to CH	0.0950	0.0608	0.00570

[1] SEM = pooled standard error of means; Means with the different letter within the same row are significantly different ($P < 0.05$).

[2] Peak center for the carbonyl ester (C=O) stretching vibration band was ca. 1740 cm^{-1}; baseline ca. 1770-1725 cm^{-1}

3. Discriminating and Classifying Structural Differences in Antisymmetric and Symmetric CH3 and CH2 Region and Carbonyl C=O Ester Region: Comparison Between Varieties

3.1. Multivariate Molecular Spectral Analyses

Two multivariate molecular spectral analyses, hierarchical cluster analysis (CLA) and principal components analysis (PCA) (Yu 2005; 2008), were used to compare the original spectra of green-type and yellow type of CDC peas to determine underlying structural differences between varieties.

For hierarchical cluster analysis (CLA) and principal components analysis (PCA), two lipid related spectral regions were used. The 1st one is the spectral region at ca. 3001-2799 cm^{-1} showing C-H function groups: CH_3 antisymmetric stretching vibration band, CH_2 antisymmetric stretching vibration band, CH_3 symmetric stretching vibration band, and CH_2 symmetric stretching vibration band. The 2nd one is the spectral region at ca. 1771-1714 cm^{-1} showing carbonyl C=O ester band that are mainly associated with lipid biopolymers in CDC peas. The spectra were used in this study without smoothing and parameterization. No FSD spectra or the 2nd derivative spectra were applied (Yu, 2011).

Hierarchical cluster analysis can be used to cluster spectra based on similarity with other spectra. Hierarchical cluster analysis (CLA) results were presented as dendograms while principal components analysis (PCA) results were plotted based on the first two highest factor scores and plotted as a function of those scores. In each comparison the eigenvector for PC1 was plotted against that of PC2 which accounted for over 90 of the variability in the spectral data of green and yellow CDC peas.

For multivariate analyses, little time is needed for this analysis. The benefit of cluster analysis is that no other prior knowledge of the sample other than a spectrum is required to make a possible distinction (Doiron et al., 2009; Yu, 2011). In this study, multivariate spectral analyses were performed using Statistica 8.0 software (StatSoft Inc, Tulsa, OK, USA).

3.2. Discriminating and Classifying Structural Differences between Raw Green-Type (CDC Strike) and Raw Yellow-Type (CDC Meadow)

The implications of the multivariate analyses are that with a pool of spectra we only need to analyze an unknown spectrum of interest to discover whether technologically processed plant-based food or feed samples are similar to the untreated ones (Doiron et al., 2009a,b). In this study, the Ward's algorithm method was used in CLA analysis without any prior parameterization of the spectral data (original anti-symmetric and symmetric CH_3 and CH_2 spectral data) in the two regions (ca. 3001-2799 cm^{-1}; ca. 1771-1714 cm^{-1}). PCA analysis was applied to identify the main sources of variation in the same two regions to identify features that differed between these cultivars and treatments.

Figures 4 (c,d) clear shows that two classes can be distinguished in the region of ca. 1771-1714 cm^{-1} based on 1st PC between raw Green-Type (CDC Strike) and raw Yellow-Type (CDC Meadow), indicating that the structure associated with lipid carbonyl C=O ester differ between the green-type and yellow-type of pea varieties. Figure 4 (a,b) also shows that separate classes in the region of ca. 3001-2799 cm^{-1} can be distinguished based on 2nd PC between the green-type and yellow-type of pea varieties indicating that the structures associated with lipid related anti-symmetric and symmetric CH_3 and CH_2 differ between the green-type and yellow-type of pea varieties.

3. Conclusion, Implications and Future Research

In conclusion, there were no difference in spectral profiles of lipid biopolymer structure conformation between raw green-type (cv. CDC Strike) and yellow-type (cv. CDC Meadow) of CDC pea varieties. The implication of this study is that the internal structural of feed and food could be detected on a molecular basis within intact tissue without destroying the inherent structure which usually damaged by wet-chemical lab processing and digestion.

I: Raw Green-Type (CDC Strike) vs. Raw-Yellow Type (CDC Meadow Peas) in anti-symmetric and symmetric CH_3 and CH_2 region

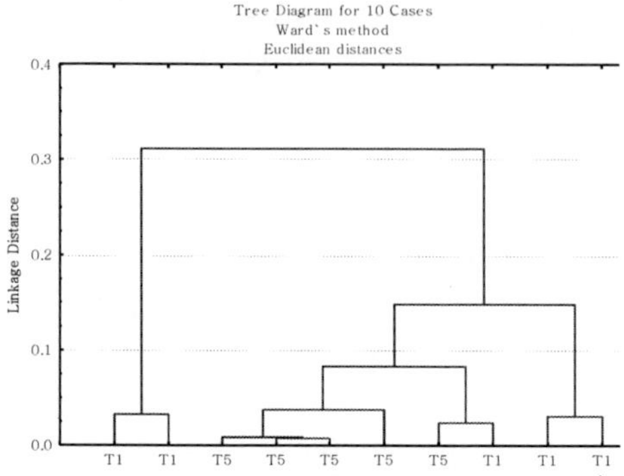

(a) Cluster analysis of spectra: CDC Strike (code = T1) vs. CDC Meadow (code = T5) in the anti-symmetric and symmetric CH_3 and CH_2 region 3001-2799 cm-1

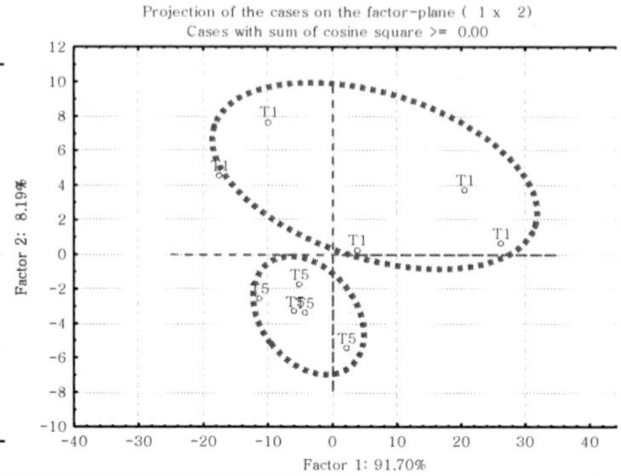

(b) Principal component analysis: CDC Strike (code = T1) vs. CDC Meadow (code = T5) in the anti-symmetric and symmetric CH_3 and CH_2 region 3001-2799 cm-1: 1st vs. 2nd PC

II: Raw Green Type (CDC Strike) vs. Raw Yellow Type (CDC Meadow Peas) in carbonyl ester C=O band region

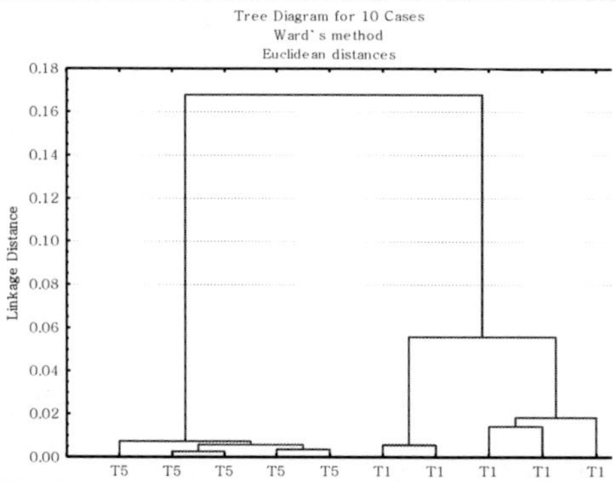

c) Cluster analysis of spectra: CDC Strike (code = T1) vs. CDC Meadow (code = T5) in the carbonyl ester C=O band region 1771-1714 cm-1

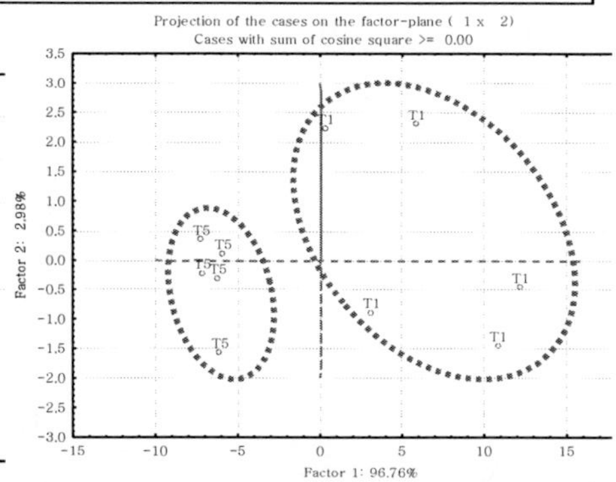

(d) Principal component analysis: CDC Strike (code = T1) vs. CDC Meadow (code = T5) in the carbonyl ester C=O band region 1771-1714 cm-1;1st vs. 2nd principal component

Figure 4. Multivariate spectral analyses of the anti-symmetric and symmetric CH_2 and CH_3 region of ca. 3001-2799 cm-1 (I) and carbonyl ester C=O band region of ca. 1771-1714 cm-1 (II) regions between raw green type (CDC Strike) vs. raw yellow type (CDC Meadow) of peas: a) & c) left columns: CLA cluster with Distance method: Euclidean; Cluster method: Ward's algorithm); b) & d) right columns: PCA analyses.

Future study is needed on the response and sensitivities to various processing application in the protein, structural and non-strucutral carbohydrate related functional groups to see how they response to different processing methods and how structural changes affect the nutrient value.

ACKNOWLEDGMENTS

Our research programs have been supported by the Ministry of Agriculture Strategic Research Chair Program, Saskatchewan Agricultural Development Fund, Natural Sciences and Engineering Research Council of Canada (NSERC, Individual Discovery Grant and CRD grant) etc. The authors thank Professor Dr. Tom Warkentin (Crop Development Centre (CDC, University of Saskatchewan, Canada) for providing the CDC samples.

REFERENCES

Doiron, K.J., Yu, P., McKinnon, J.J, Christensen, D.A. 2009a. Heat-induced protein structures and protein subfractions in relation to protein degradation kinetics and intestinal availability in dairy cattle. *J. Dairy Sci.* 92, 3319-3330.

Doiron, K.J., Yu, P., Christensen, C.R., Christensen, D.A., McKinnon, J.J. 2009b. Detecting molecular changes in Vimy flaxseed protein structure using synchrotron FTIRM and DRIFT spectroscopic techniques: Structural and biochemical characterization. Spectroscopy. 23, 307–322

Goelema, J.O., 1999. Processing of legume seeds: effect on digestive behavious in dairy cows. Ph.D Thesis. Wageningen Agricultural University, The Netherlands.

Himmelsbach, D.S., Khalili, S., Akin, D.E. 1998. FT-IR microspectroscopic imaging of flax (linum usitatissimum L.) stems. *Cell. Mol. Bio.* 44, 99-108.

Jonker, A., Gruber, M.Y., Wang, Y., McKinnon, J.J., Colman, B., Christensen, D.A., Yu, P. 2012. Foam stability of leaves from anthocyanidin-accumulating Lc-alfalfa and relation to molecular structures detected by fourier-transformed infrared-vibration spectroscopy. *Grass and Forage Science*. 67, 369-381.

Khan, M.M.R., Yu, P. 2013. Document Thermal stability and molecular microstructure of heat-induced cereal grains, revealed with Raman molecular microspectroscopy and differential scanning calorimetry. *J. Agric. Food Chem.* 61, 6495-6504.

Marinkovic, N.S., Chance, M.R. 2006. Synchotron Infared Microscopy, Encyclopedia of Molecular Cell Biology and Molecular Me*dicine*, 2nd Ed., Vol. 13, R. Meyers, Editor, Wiley Inc., pp. 671-708.

Peng, Q., Khan, N.A., Wang, Z., Yu, P. 2014. Moist and dry heating-induced changes in protein molecular structure, protein subfractions, and nutrient profiles in camelina seeds. *J. Dairy Sci.* 97, 446-457.

Samadi, P. Yu. 2011. Determine heat-induced changes of protein molecular structure, protein subfraction and nutrient profiles in soybean seeds affected dry and moisture heat processing. *J. Dairy Sci.* 94, 6092-6102.

The Western Producer. 2014. New green pea varieties could soon be available. Available on Web on May 31, 2014.

Warkentin, T., Vandenberg, A., Tar'an, B., Banniza, S., Barlow, B., I. Scott. 2009. CDC Meadow field pea. *Can. J. Plant Sci.* 87: 909–910.

Walhain, P., Foucart, M., Thewis, A., 1992. Influence of extrusion on ruminal and intestinal disappearance *in sacco* of pea proteins and starch. *Anim. Feed Sci. Technol.* 38, 43-55.

Wetzel, D.L., Eilert, A.J., Pietrzak, L.N., Miller, S.S., Sweat, J.A. 1998. Ultraspatially resolved synchrotron infrared microspectroscopy of plant tissue in situ. *Cell. Mol. Bio.* 44, 145-167.

Yu, P., J.O. Goelema, B.J. Leury, S. Tamminga and A.R. Egan. 2002. An analysis of the nutritive value of heat processed legume seeds for animal production using the DVE/OEB model: A review. *Anim. Feed Sci. Technol.* 99 (1-4): 141-176.

Yu, P. 2004. Application of advanced synchrotron-based Fourier transform infrared microspectroscopy (SR-FTIR) to animal nutrition and feed science: a novel approach. *Br. J. Nutr.* 92, 869-885

Yu, P., Tamminga, S., Egan, A.R., Christensen, D.A. 2004a. Probing equivocal effects of heat processing of legume seeds on performance of ruminants - A review. Asian-Australasian J. Anim. Sci. 17, 869-876.

Yu, P. 2005. *Application of cluster analysis (CLA) in feed chemical imaging to accurately reveal structural-chemical features of feeds within cellular dimension. J. Agric. Food Chem.* 53, 2872-2880.

Yu, P. 2005. Applications of hierarchical cluster analysis (CLA) and principal component analysis (PCA) in feed structure and feed molecular chemistry research, using synchrotron-based Fourier transform infrared (FTIR) microspectroscopy. *J. Agric. Food Chem.* 53, 7115-7127.

Yu, P. 2008. Synchrotron-based microspectroscopic analysis of molecular and biopolymer structures using multivariate techniques and advanced multi-components modeling. *Can. J. Analytical Sci. Spectroscopy.* 53, 220-231.

Yu, P. 2010. *Book Chapter 27. Detect Structural Features of Asymmetric and Symmetric CH2 and CH3 Functional Groups and Their Ratio of Biopolymers within Intact Tissue in Complex Plant System Using Synchrotron FTIRM and DRIFT Molecular Spectroscopy.* In: Biopolymers; ISBN 978-953-307-109-1; Editor: Professor Dr. Magdy M. Elnashar; pp 535-546.

Yu, P. 2010. *Plant-Based Food and Feed Protein Structure Changes Induced by Gene-Transformation, Heating and Bio-Ethanol Processing: A Novel Synchrotron-Based Molecular Structure and Nutrition Research Program. Molecular Nutrition and Food Research* (MNF). 54, 1535–1545.

Yu, P. 2011. Study the sensitivity of molecular functional groups to bioethanol processing in lipid biopolymer of co-products using DRIFT molecular spectroscopy. Spectrochimica Acta - Part A: *Molecular and Biomolecular Spectroscopy*, 82, 1-7.

Yu, P. 2012. Book Chapter 5. Peas (*Pisum sativum*): Chemical, Molecular Structural, Biodegradation and Nutritional Characterization, In: Peas: Cultivation, Varieties and Nutritional Uses; ISBN 978-1-61942-866-9/978-1-61942-886-7; Editor: Aiden M. Comstock and Braylen E. Lothrop; pp125-142. Published by *Nova Science Publishers,* Inc. New York. USA.

In: *Pisum sativum*
Editor: Shannell Becket
ISBN: 978-1-63463-230-0

Chapter 6

ACYRTHOSIPHON PISUM (HARRIS) PUSHES COOL-SEASON FOOD LEGUMES TO EXTINCTION IN ETHIOPIA

Melaku Wale*
Bahir Dar University, Bahir Dar, Ethiopia

ABSTRACT

This review summarizes studies carried out on pea aphids, *Acyrtosiphon pisum* (Harris) (Aphididae: Homoptera) damaging food legumes in northwestern Ethiopia (much of the high plateau of the country is found here, over 2000 m above sea level) from 1998 to 2013. The review summarizes of various papers on pea aphids published in the area of wild legumes, aphid reproduction and survival, population dynamics, suitable weather conditions, host preference and evaluation of eco-friendly botanical products against aphids. During the initial studies, we tried to identify how aphids over winter the rather long (9-month) dry season. It was found that wild leguminous plants such as clover, *Trifolium ruepellainum* and vetch, *Vicia* spp and the cultivated ones such as the perennial legumes (pigeon pea, *Cajanus cajan*) served as wild hosts. These are believed to sustain aphid survival during the dry season. In the greenhouse study, it was determined that the more the aphid

*Email: melakuwale@gmail.com

density the lower the rate of reproduction and the longevity of aphids. Aphid population dynamics studies also showed that aphids prefer cool and dry climate, nevertheless warm episodes are necessary for reproduction. Lower altitudes are therefore found good hot-spots for the aphids. Our research station (Adet Research Center, Amhara, Ethiopia) is located at 2240 m a.s.l. where the aphids are less important while 45 km north the altitude descends 400 m lower than our station, gets warmer and grass pea production has almost stopped there because of these aphids. Aphid numbers steadily increased from seedling stage to pod setting, and then drastically fell at maturity. Lentils and grass peas were more suitable hosts than faba bean and field pea. In Ethiopia, pea aphids were first reported in cool and dry regions of the extreme north, which later extended their range to even lower altitudes and warmer areas. Management studies carried out include botanicals, detergents, kerosene and some of the more conventional and aphid-specific pesticides. Promising botanicals included spray of capsicum juice, kerosene (despite its phytotoxicity) and detergents. Parasitism of aphids by *Aphidius* species and predation by coccinellid larvae and adults was high but they came late long after damage was inflicted to the crop. The series of studies carried out over the years helped to determine the status of the pest in the area and point out some of the environmentally safe management options. Planting susceptible legumes may have to be limited to places where the aphid is not endemic or better use aphid-specific pesticides (such as pirimicarb). Spraying alternate hosts during the off-season to break the cycle of infestation, determining the rate and frequency of botanicals such as capsicum, and ensuring the survival of coccinellids and aphid parasitoids during the offseason can be the next research agenda.

1. INTRODUCTION

The cool-season food legumes are important grain products in Ethiopia. Field pea (*Pisum sativum* L.), faba bean (*Vicia faba* L.), lentil (*Lens culinaris* Medik.) and grass pea (*Lathyrussativus* L.) are the most important ones. The Ethiopian highland plateau is suitable for these cool season legumes because it mimics the more temperate climate of the Mediterranean region where most of these legumes are believed to have originated. Ethiopia is believed to be the second largest faba bean producer in the world only after China (Abebe et al., 2014). Because most people in Ethiopia cannot afford animal protein, legumes have long constituted their protein diets for millennia.

However, these grain crops are not without constraints in the country. The pea aphid, *Acyrthosiphon pisum* (Harris) (Aphididae: Homoptera), among others, is a major pest that is pushing pulses out of production. It feeds on a wide range of plants that belong to 14 genera, the major ones being *Coronilla, Lens, Lotus, Medicago, Melilotus, Pisum, and Vigna* (Ellsbury and Nielson, 1981). Pea aphids attack all kinds of peas (garden and field peas) (*Pisum sativum*), alfalfa (*Medicago sativa*), clover (*Trifolium* sp.), and other leguminous crops except those in the genus Phaseolus (Ellsbury and Nielson, 1981; Davidson and Lyon, 1987). Lucerne (*Medicago sativa),* pea *(Pisumsativum),* clover *(Trifoliumruepellanium),* egg-plant *(Solannum melongena),* vetch *(Vicia* spp*) and* broad bean *(Vicia fabae)* are heavily attacked (Archibald, 1979). It infests Lucerne to such an extent that the ground turns white due to exuviae (Archibald, 1979).

In addition to the irreversible damage due to direct plant sap sucking, pea aphids transmit viral diseases that cause total crop loss. Losses in the production of peas probably exceed that caused by any other pest of peas (Davidson and Lyon, 1987).

Pea aphid is distributed throughout North America (Davidson and Lyon, 1987), Europe, Asia and the cooler areas of East Africa (Autrique et al., 1989). Host variety and aphid biotype are important for the host and aphid association (Bournoville et al., 2000; Caillaud and Via, 2000; Morgan et al., 2001).

Prior to 1983 when Crowe and Ali (1983) published a checklist of 64 species of aphids recorded in Ethiopia, *A. pisum* was reported but was not considered important. Abate et al. (1982) and Ali and Gebremedhin (1990) have reported its minor pest status in earlier surveys in Ethiopia. Nevertheless, the pest has quickly become a key pest of legumes since 1983/84 season (Ali and Gebremedhin, 1990). Ever since it has been widening its geographical coverage and the range of plant species attacked.

In Ethiopia, the pea aphid has a holocyclic life cycle, i.e., it reproduces parthenogentically without producing sexual forms, which is typical of tropical and subtropical species (Cardona et al., 1984; Ali and Gebremedhin, 1990). Viviparity permits rapid exploitation of the host plant as its parthenogenetic multiplication rate, without fertilization, is potentially enormous. In temperate areas, pea aphids reproduce both sexually (via eggs) during the winter and parthenogenetically during the summer (Davidson and Lyon, 1987).

Yield loss caused by pea aphids on field pea can be as high as 37% at some regions (Gebremedhin, 1990). To date, total (100%) crop failures have become common in many parts of Ethiopia (Andarge and Berhan, 1998). Growers in Zema valley of West Gojam zone, Ethiopia, for example, have quit field pea cultivation due to pea aphids and shifted to haricot bean production, a recently introduced leguminous crop of the *Phaseolus* genus. Total crop failure of grass pea is commonplace near Bahir Dar, Ethiopia (M. Wale, Pers. Obs.). Here, farmers harvest the grain-less crop as livestock feed.

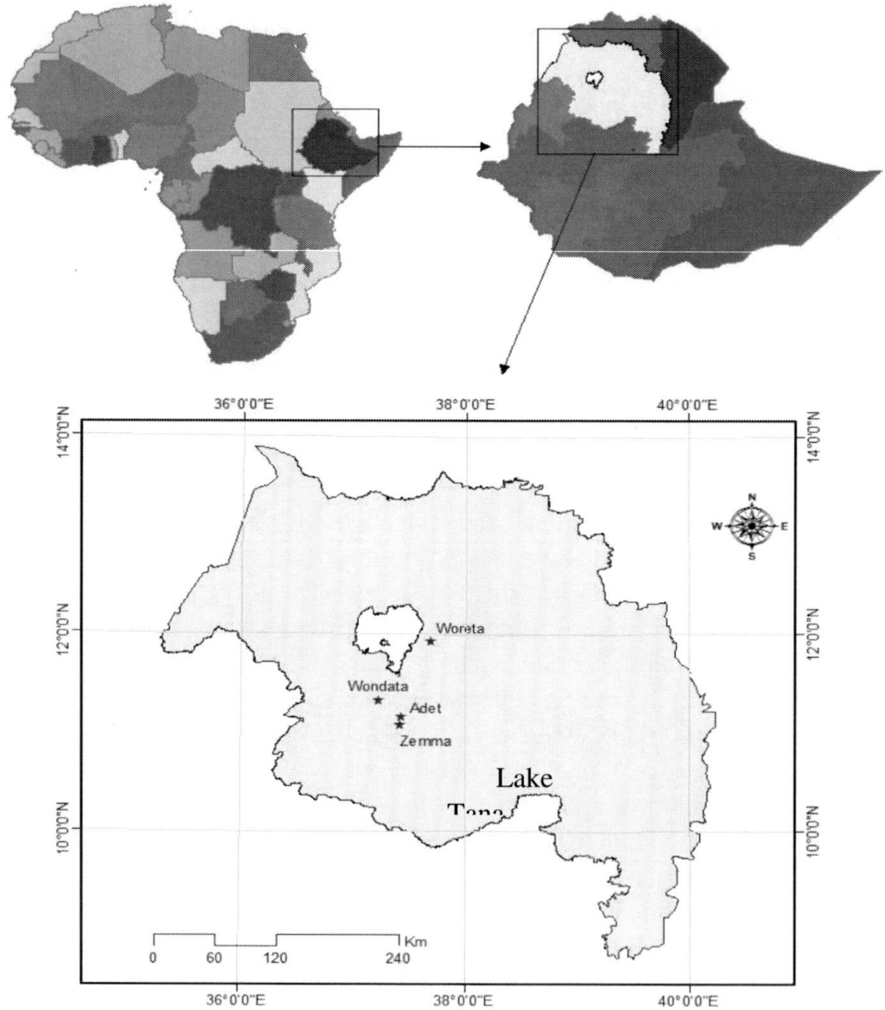

Figure 1. Map showing the study areas in northwestern Ethiopia (Amhara region).

The Amhara Agricultural Research Institute, Ethiopia, is a public institute dedicated to improve the quality of life of the farming community in Ethiopia and beyond through science and technology. Bahir Dar University is one of the seven universities in the Amhara State, Ethiopia, which participated in some of the latest studies reviewed. The current review reports major findings of a series of studies carried out on pea aphids in northwestern Ethiopia from 1989 to 2012 (Figure 1).

2. THE STUDY REGION

The State of Amhara of Ethiopia encompasses two ecologically distinct regions, i.e., western Amhara and eastern Amhara. The study area is situated in western Amhara, which is also known as north-western Ethiopia, the area where studies for the current review is based. This area itself is topographically divided into two main parts, namely the highlands and lowlands. The highlands are above 1500 meters above sea level and comprise the largest part of the northern and eastern parts of the region. The highlands are also characterized by chains of mountains and plateaus. Ras Dejen (4620 m), the highest peak in the country, Guna (4236 m), Choke (4184 m) and Abune – Yousef (4190 m) are among the mountain peaks that are located in the highland parts of the region. The lowland part covers mainly the extreme western and eastern parts of the region with an altitude between 500-1500 meters above sea level. The annual mean temperature for most parts of the region lies between 15°C-21°C. The State receives the highest percentage (80%) of the total rainfall in the country. The highest rainfall occurs during the summer season, which starts in mid June and ends in early September. The publications reviewed here were carried out near Lake Tana, the largest lake in the country, 4 thousand km^2 area, the source of the Blue Nile River, which then becomes the international river Nile. The studies were carried out in ecologically distinct areas around Lake Tana, i.e., Zemma, Adet, Wondata and Woreta (Figure 1). Faba bean and field pea are grown on well drained loam soils and grass pea and lentil on dense black soils on residual moisture. Wondata and Woreta are black soil dominated, Adet red soil and Zemma intermediate. Laboratory studies were carried out at Adet.

3. Biology and Ecology

a. Number of Molts (Instars)

In a study carried out in the greenhouse (ambient temperature and humidity) to determine the growth and development of pea aphids on various legumes, the number of molts did not vary between legume species (faba bean also called broad bean, field pea, lentil and grass pea) (Wale et al., 2000). The study also indicated that in northwestern Ethiopia, under experimental conditions, the pea aphid undergoes up to three molts. This indicates the number of nymphal stages. The nymphal period lasted between nine and 11 days and did not vary among legumes. It appears that the warm episodes in the area speed up maturity of pea aphids. Similar findings were reported elsewhere (Sharma et al., 1976).

b. Adult Longevity and Fecundity

Lifespan. The lifespan of the pea aphid, from birth to death, was significantly longer on lentil than on other crops (Wale et al., 2000). Pea aphids lived for about a month on lentil, with their lifespan ranging from 27 to 41. Pea aphid lifespan was 20.1 days on faba bean, 22.7 on field pea, 34.9 on lentil and 24.6 on grass pea. Extended reproductive and post-reproductive period of pea aphid on lentil resulted in longer lifespan. The shortest lifespan was recorded on faba bean with a mean of about 20 and a range of 15- to 26 days (Table 1).

Survival curve. Slightly more pea aphids survived on field pea for the first 10 days of adult life after which more aphids survived on lentil than all other crops (Wale et al., 2000). The shortest survival duration of all ages of the aphid was recorded on faba bean. Aphids survived on this host for 17 days. Pea aphids survived less on faba bean and better on lentils and field pea.

Adult life history. Significantly higher reproductive period, post-reproductive period and longevity of pea aphids were recorded on lentil than on other crops (Wale et al., 2000). This is in agreement with lifespan and survival curves mentioned above (Table 1).

Table 1. Duration (in days) of different periods of adult stage of the pea aphid on four cultivated legumes in northwestern Ethiopia in 1998 and 1999*

Crop species	Period in days (days ± SE, N)			
	Pre-reproductive period**	Reproductive	Post-reproductive**	Longevity
Faba bean	0.9±0.1, 10 b	9.8±1.0, 10 c	1.0±0.1, 10 b	11.1±1.3, 10 c
Field pea	1.2±0.1, 10 a	9.8±0.6, 10 c	1.3±0.2, 10 b	22.7±1.5, 10 bc
Lentil	1.1±0.1, 9 a	17.4±0.9, 9 a	2.1±0.3, 9 b	25.2±1.5, 9 a
Grass pea	0.9±0.1, 9 ab	14.3±1.2, 9 b	0.7±0.0, 9 b	15.3±1.0, 9 b

*Mean separation by least significant difference test, α=0.05; means followed by different letters within a column are significantly different from each other; **Square root transformed values using the formula $\sqrt{(x+0.5)}$ where x indicates original values of duration in days. The original values of pre-reproductive and post-reproductive period were more variable than reproductive period and longevity and they required square root transformation to stabilize variance. N stands for number of aphids tested.

c. Lifetime Fecundity

*Basic life table parameters.*Whereas net reproductive rate was highest on lentil (103.6 females/female), the rates of population increase was highest on faba bean due the shorter generation time on it (Wale et al., 2000) (Table 2). The second highest rate of population increase and reproductive rate was observed on grass pea. The pea aphid doubled its population in less than three days on all four crop species. The shortest pre-reproductive period was recorded on faba bean.

Lifetime fecundity of the pea aphid was higher on lentil than on the other crop species tested, followed by grass pea, faba bean and field pea (Table 3). Pea aphids developing on lentil produced an average of 115 and on grass pea 83 nymphs. Pea aphids reared on faba bean and field pea had significantly lower nymphal production than the other two. The difference in lifetime fecundity was caused by higher daily reproduction on lentil (Table 3).

Table 2. Life table parameters for *A. pisum* reared on different food legumes

	Net reproductive rate (R_o)	Mean generation time (days)	Intrinsic rate of increase (r)	Doubling time (days)
Faba bean	59.40	14.27	0.286	2.42
Field pea	62.59	16.04	0.256	2.69
Lentil	103.56	18.07	0.257	2.70
Grass pea	82.90	16.02	0.276	2.51

*Mean separation by least significant difference test, α=0.05; **Square root transformed values using the formula $\sqrt{(x+0.5)}$ where *x* indicates original values of duration in days. The original values of pre-reproductive and post-reproductive period were more variable than reproductive period and longevity and they required square root transformation to stabilize variance.

Table 3. Life-time fecundity and mean daily reproduction of *A.pisum* reared on different food legumes

Crop species	Reproduction (Nymphs/ female±SE, N)	Range	Number of nymphs: Number/day/female (Nymphs±SE, N)	Range
Faba bean	59.7±5.8, 10 c	35-89	6.2±1.8, 10 ab	1-9
Field pea	57.9±4.0, 10 c	42-86	5.3±0.9, 10 b	0-8
Lentil	115.1±5.3, 9 b	89-145	6.7±0.6, 9 a	0-12
Grass pea	82.9±7.7, 9 b	35-127	5.4±0.9, 9 b	1-8

*Mean separation by least significant difference test, α=0.05; means followed by different letters within a column are significantly different from each other.

Reproductive curve. Pea aphids produced more nymphs per day on lentil than on other crops (Wale et al., 2000). The peak daily nymphal production was recorded from adults aged between 6 and 10 days. Reproduction continued for 21 days on lentil, 19 days on grass pea, 18 days on field pea and 16 days on faba bean. After a break of about one week, reproduction on lentil resumed, and produced a small second peak between 27 and 30 days of adult age. On other crops there was no second peak and daily reproduction progressively declined until it reached nil. The mean daily reproduction of pea aphids, obtained by dividing the total number of nymphs produced per aphid by the number of days the aphid produced the nymphs, was significantly higher on lentil, followed by faba bean. Differences among the rest of the host plants were not significant. A maximum of 12 nymphs/day was recorded on lentil, 9 on field pea and faba bean, and 8 on grass pea. This indicates that the pea aphid varies in its daily reproduction due to differences in host plant and here lentil is more susceptible to damage by pea aphids than are field pea, grass pea and faba bean. Similar differences have been reported on other leguminous plants elsewhere (Kaakeh and Ducther, 1993).

Effect of minimum and maximum temperatures on aphid survival and reproduction was computed. Significant relationship was obtained between daily nymphal production and minimum temperature on lentil alone ($F=4.61$, $P<0.05$). The relationship of aphid survival and minimum temperature was also nearly significant ($F=4.07$, $P=0.06$). There was no discernible relationship between survival/reproduction and maximum temperature.

4. Wild and Cultivated Hosts of Pea Aphid

These are legumes (perennial or annual) that grow wild or are cultivated for fodder or for other purposes. They do not belong to food-legumes. We found clover (wild), vetch and pigeon pea (cultivated) that are infested by pea aphids.

In a field survey carried out in 1999 and 2000 in West Gojam, northwestern Ethiopia, wild or cultivated annual and perennial legume plants were sampled for the presence of pea aphids on 0.5×0.5 m^2 quadrates which were selected randomly (Wale et al., 2003a).

In case of annual plants, pea aphids infested vetches (*Vicia* spp.) and clover (*Trifolium ruepellanium* Fresen) significantly ($\chi^2=245.7$, $P=0.005$). This was not found to be the case on lupine (*Lupinus* spp.) and alfalfa (*Medicago sativa* L.). Aphids infested flowers of clover, and flowers, leaves, and stems of vetch. Despite the search for its existence on many perennial trees, pea aphid was consistently found only on the perennial pigeon pea (*Cajanus cajan*) plants throughout the year and not on others such as sesbania, *Sesbania sesban* (L.) Merr.

Clover plants were found growing in pasturelands and as undergrowth beneath large cereals such as maize and sorghum or even under small cereals such as wheat and barley. Clover plants were found infested more in October when the plants flowered and set pods as compared to other times of the year (Wale et al., 2003a). From December onwards, these plants almost disappeared except in very wet conditions such as near leaking water taps, irrigation channels and stream banks. Clover plant density and aphid numbers declined through to January and February. Vetch plants, on the other hand, were found infested a bit earlier than clover, i.e, in September.

Pea aphid density varied significantly between the different legumes (Wale et al., 2003a). Vetch plants carried more aphid load per plant than clover in all survey areas (χ^2=10.2, P=0.005, df=1). Furthermore, vetch plants in the forage field were carrying more aphid load than vetch plants in the crop field margin.

Literature indicates that low protein to sugar ratio of plants contributes for immunity to pea aphids (Nielsen and Lehman, 1980). Pea aphids choose plants with more protein levels. This may, among other factors such as biotype specificity to specific varieties, have contributed for the absence of aphids on alfalfa. In the present study, lupines were found immune to aphids; alkaloids in lupine may have served as deterrents. Studies in Poland have shown it is the alkaloids in the phloem sap of lupine plants that determine their resistance to attack by pea aphid (Wegorek and Krzymanska, 1975). One other reason may be that the aphid biotypes present in Ethiopia may have evolved specifically adapted to the pulses grown in Ethiopia for a long time in the past.

5. Reproduction and Survival

The effect of pea aphid density (2, 6, 10 and 14 nymphs/per plant) on survival and reproduction was studied on four cool-season food legumes, i.e., on faba bean, field pea, lentil and grass pea in the greenhouse in northwestern Ethiopia at ambient temperature and humidity. Aphid survival generally tended to decline with increasing aphid density per plant particularly on faba bean (Wale et al., 2003b). Decline was more consistent with grass pea, perhaps because it was the source of the test aphids that were used in the study. Aphid stock cultures were prepared by using aphids from grass peas widely grown in the area. Aphids survived significantly longer on lentil when 2 aphids were allowed to feed on a plant compared to when 6, 10 and 14 aphids per plant were allowed (Wale et al., 2003b) (Figure 2).

Similarly, progeny production consistently declined with increasing aphid density per plant on the four crops (Wale et al., 2003b). Low aphid density, i.e., 2 aphids/ plant, gave the highest mean progeny production, i.e., 37.3 offspring/female, regardless of legume species. Again regardless of density, the number of nymphs produced per aphid was significantly lower on faba bean compared to the other host plants, indicating unsuitability of faba bean for pea aphid survival and reproduction.

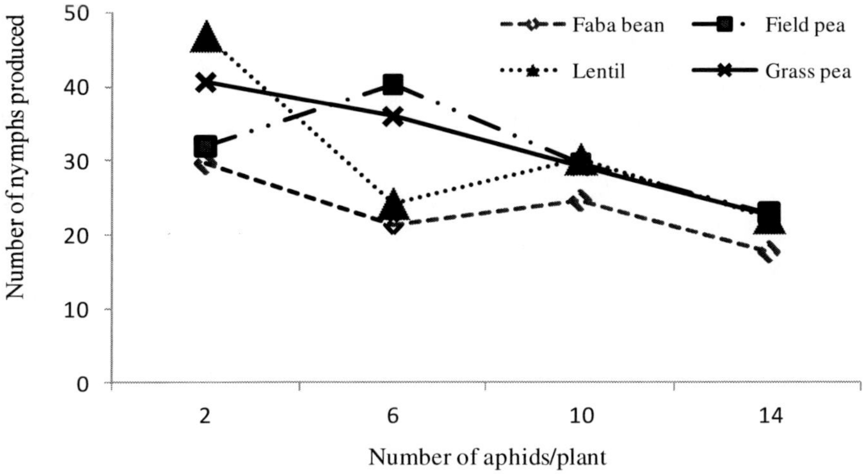

Figure 2. Number of nymphs produced per aphid at various aphid densities per plant on four legumes.

On the other hand, daily nymphal production was significantly affected by aphid density per plant. On faba bean, 2 aphids/ plant gave the highest daily reproduction, while 14 aphids/ plant had the lowest. Reproduction showed a decreasing trend as aphid density increased in all test crop species. For all aphid densities, reproduction started to decline after 8 days on each of faba bean and grass pea, after 6 days on field pea and lentil (Wale et al., 2003b).

6. Population Dynamics

Basic estimates of populations are required in integrated pest management in order to understand the population dynamics of a pest species and as the basis for making management decisions relating to monitoring and forecasting levels of pest abundance and distribution (Dent, 2000). Absolute estimates of aphids per unit plant were recorded.

The population dynamics of pea aphids was investigated on field peas at two locations: Adet (relatively cooler area at 2240 m altitude) and Zema (warmer and lower than 2000 m altitude) for three years (seasons), i.e., 1994, 1995 and 1996.

The cooler location is located at 11° 17' N latitude and 37°43' longitudes on an altitude of 2240 m above sea level. The center receives average annual rainfall of 1271 mm and temperature ranging from 8.8-25.2^{o}C (ARC, 2011).

Planting was staggered to mimic growers' practice. In contrast to the lower altitude area, pea aphid numbers per plant increased as planting was delayed (Wale, 2002).

At the cooler location, a total of 8 thousand aphids were recorded in 1995, 5 thousand in 1994 and 4 thousand in 1996. At the warmer location, between 10 thousand and 12 thousand aphids were counted during the same period. This indicates that aphids always need warm temperature to speed up their reproduction (Wale, 2002).

At the cooler location, the peaks of weekly aphid numbers were high in August; and the seasonal totals of aphid populations increased as planting time was delayed. At the warmer location, it was difficult to discern peaks because they varied with season. Peaks were observed in July, early and mid September depending on season.

Number of natural enemies (predators such as coccinellids and parasitoids such as *Aphidius* spp.) varied with season (year); they were more in 1996 than other years (Wale et al., 2002).

Coccinellids can prevent overpopulation of aphids and their harmful effects; however, the population of aphids is reduced only after damage is inflicted to the crop (Hodek, 1967). Without natural enemies, aphid numbers quickly reach very high proportions. Parasitoids/predators recorded so far on pea aphid in Ethiopia include *Aphidius (?) urticae*, *Cheilomenes lunata* and *C. sulphurea* (Abate, 1991). The different events in the life history of aphids are shown on Figure 3.

Generally weekly aphid populations showed positive correlation with ambient maximum temperature, but negative correlation with ambient minimum temperature and relative humidity. Increasing maximum temperature promoted the buildup of aphid populations while increased minimum temperature, increased rainfall and relative humidity suppressed it. As planting was delayed, grain yield increased at the cooler location; it decreased at the warmer place. This happened because early planted plots suffered from severe storm damage while the late one did not. From these results, it is recommended that planting of field peas should take place from mid- to late June at the cooler and during the first week of June at the warmer place to obtain higher yields; by doing so a mean of 0.32 t/ha more grain yield at the cooler and 0.5 t/ha at the warmer place were obtained.

In another population dynamics study carried out at Wondata (close to the Blue Nile River) and at Woreta (east of Lake Tana) on grass pea between 2009 and 2011, aphid density exponentially increased between 60 and 120 days after crop emergence and then declined starting from 135 days until harvest

(Tesfaye et al., 2012). Pea aphid density, aphid days, percent plant damage, biomass weight, and grain yield were significantly different between locations, seasons, insecticidal treatment levels and crop growth stages. Overall, 42-53% of unprotected plots and 16-20% of the protected plots showed severe symptoms of aphid damage. A maximum mean biomass yield loss of 47% and grain yield of 94% was recorded. Regression analysis of crop damage with pea aphid days was direct and significant. In contrast, regression analysis of biomass weight and grain yield with pea aphid density and pea aphid days showed significant inverse relationship.

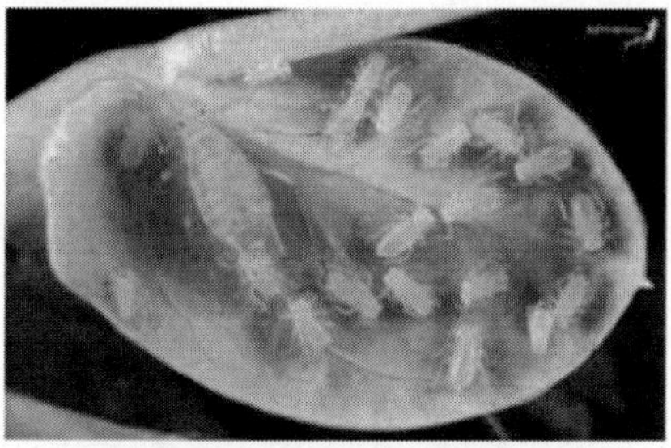

Nymph production

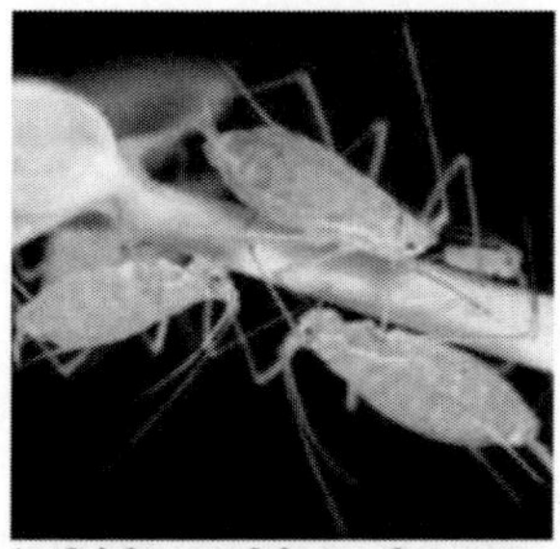

Aphids sucking plant sap

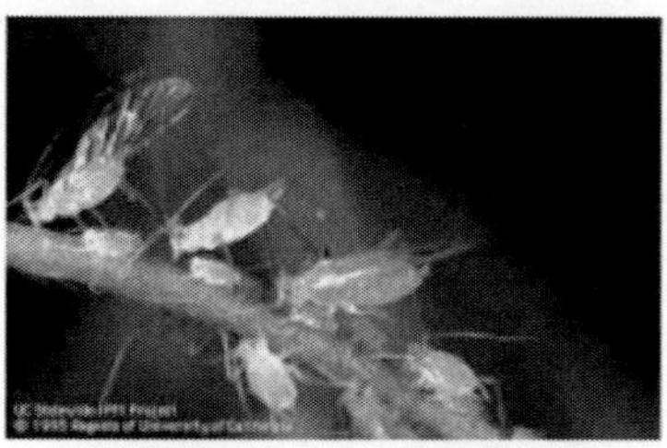

Dispersal (winged form)

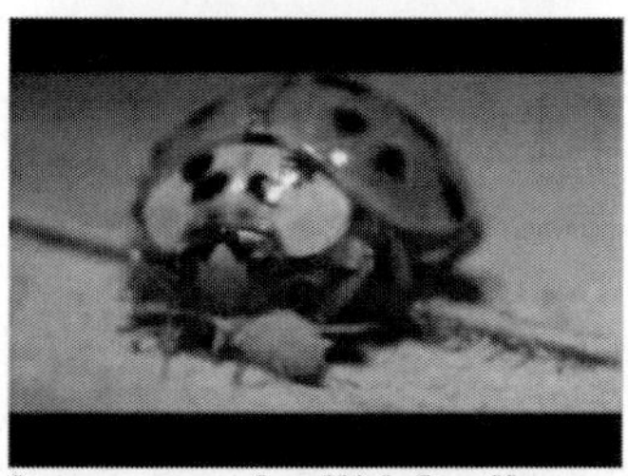

Predatory coccinellid feeding aphid

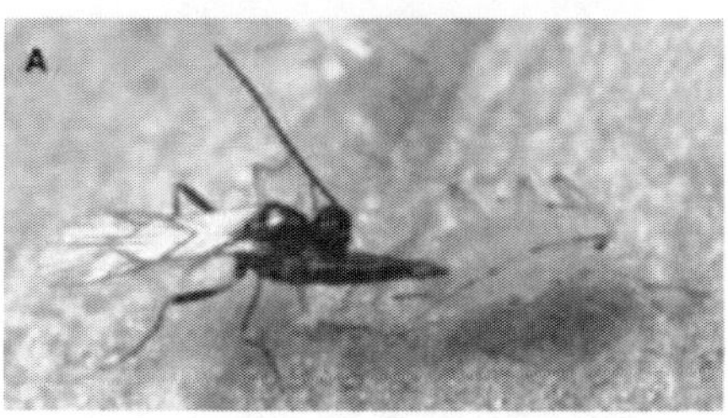

Parasitoid stinging an aphid

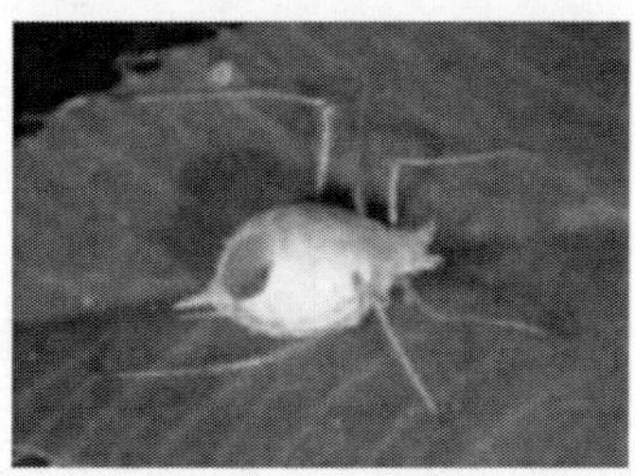

Aphid mummy (parasitoid emergence hole)

Figure 3.Different events during the life cycle of aphids. Source: various occasions and sources.

7. Host Preference

Because pea aphids severely constrain food legume production in Ethiopia, pea aphid preference and performance study on common food legumes were tested with no-choice, dual- and multiple-choice experiments under greenhouse conditions in northwestern Ethiopia.

The results revealed that pea aphids preferred field peas, lentils and grass peas more than faba bean. Growth rate of pea aphids varied with crop variety and plant growth stage. Field pea and lentils died within 30 days. Cumulative pea aphid load was higher on field pea and grass pea than on faba bean and lentil (Figure 4 and 5). In the no-choice experiment, the mean pea aphid number per five plants ranged between 1.8 at 5 days after aphid infestation (DAI) on improved faba bean and 321.5 at 20 DAI on local field pea (Tesfaye et al., 2013). In the dual- and multiple-choice experiments, aphids required less than 1 day to infest field pea, lentil and grass pea plants, and 4–11 days to infest faba bean. No variety was immune to infestation, but overall, field peas and grass peas were good hosts for culturing pea aphids. Growing susceptible crops in pea aphid hot spot areas may have to be avoided in favor of less preferred ones.

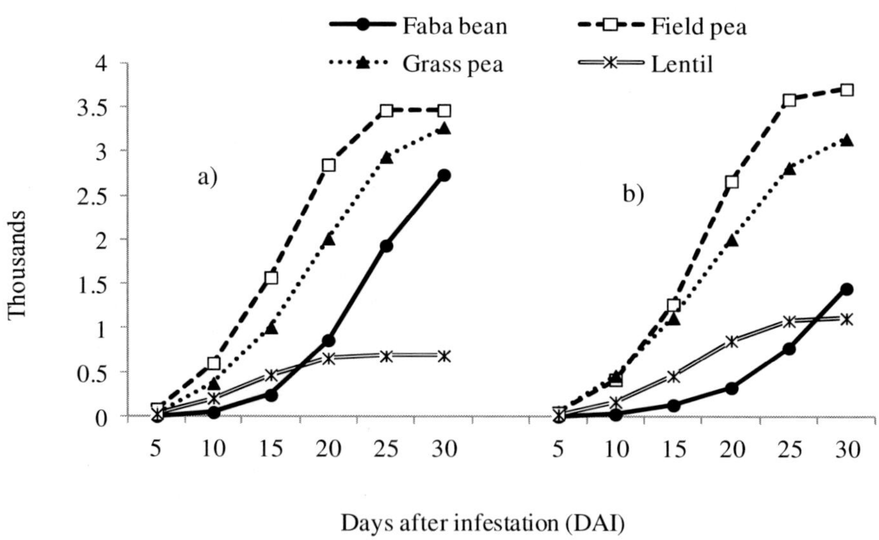

Figure 4. Cumulative pea aphid days per five plants on cool-season food legumes, a) Local varieties, b) Improved varieties.

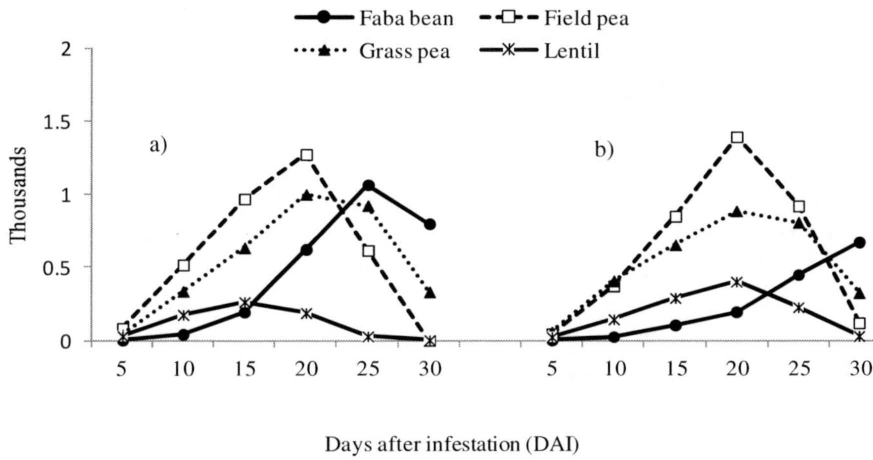

Figure 5. Mean number of pea aphids day per five plants on cool-season legumes, a) Local varieties, b) Improved varieties.

Despite the huge difference between crop types and varieties, the pea aphids successfully colonized and developed on all legumes and varieties tested. Variations were observed in the growth rate of the aphids, their colonization and preferences. All tested legume crops are recognized as hosts of pea aphids, but there was noticeable difference in preference and performance. Host plant varieties and growth stages of these crops were sources of variation for the observed difference in preference and performance of pea aphids. Aphids took long time (up to 11 days) to infest faba beans and just 1 day to infest field peas, lentils and grass peas. The population growth rate of pea aphids varied with the crop variety and growth stage. For each of the crop varieties tested, the maximum growth rate of pea aphid was 153 on local grass pea, 53 on improved grass pea, 137 on improved lentil, 112 on local field pea, 131 on improved field pea, 400 on local faba bean and 389 on improved faba bean.

Pea aphid preference and performance in dual- and multiple-choice conditions varied depending on the combination of alternative choices. For instance, lentil and field pea were found to be sensitive and died earlier under no-choice and dual-choice conditions. However, when these varieties were exposed to pea aphid with multiple choices, they sustained for long time but carried less pea aphid load. The reason behind this may be that the food availability will be higher and the pea aphid population density will be lower per plant.

The results of these greenhouse experiments should further be verified through advanced research in the laboratory (extracting secondary metabolites which favored/ disfavored pea aphids, and at molecular level) and also more field research. Moreover, the plant and the aphid side of the interaction may have to be studied for the complete understanding of the reaction of aphids on various hosts. This includes, among others, what the origin of the aphid clones are, the history of the test crops in relation to pea aphids, etc. These actions may help identify the more reliable mechanisms (chemical, physical and ecological) for the diverse interactions. None of the plants were completely avoided; pea aphid was able to build its population on all the host plants included in the study. However, its growth rate varied indicating potential for future exploitation.

8. Botanicals against Aphids

Like in many other places in Ethiopia, grass pea is grown extensively in northwestern Ethiopia, specifically at Wondata area, near the banks of the Blue Nile River. This place differs from other grass pea growing areas of Ethiopia in one point, that the crop here suffers from pea aphid infestation to the point of total loss. Grass pea is popularly known as the poor man's insurance crop, the ultimate source of protein for the poor. Grass pea growing is at the verge of collapse due to pea aphids, and although this pest can easily be stopped by chemical pesticides, these are not recommended for their drawbacks on the environment. More environment friendly and less expensive local products should be identified to replace the all too common, but effective, chemical pesticides.

Therefore, the relative efficacy of some locally available botanicals was tested against pea aphids on grass pea along with detergent, kerosene and pesticide. In search of a potentially more sustainable and environmentally friendly alternatives to the commonly used insecticides, some botanicals (neem, garlic and hot pepper), soap, kerosene, and the aphicide pirimicarb (as treated control) were tested for their efficacy against pea aphids at Wondata village, about 1 km far from the Blue Nile River, near Bahir Dar, Ethiopia from 1999 to 2002 (Wale, 2004). Juices of botanicals were sprayed on to plants at various growth stages of the crop. Next to pirimicarb, hot pepper was consistently the most effective botanical in keeping aphid numbers down and increasing the grain yield (Wale, 2004). Compared to the untreated control, pirimicarb gave 83% and hot pepper 55% less aphid population. The maximum number of aphids per 10 plants was 755, which was counted on untreated plots. Soap spray was less effective, while kerosene caused irreversible phytotoxicity. Infestation levels increased with advancing maturity of the crop, rising dramatically near crop maturity. Plant damage due to aphids was also visually assessed and the second lowest damage was recorded on hot pepper treated plots. Furthermore, pirimicarb gave 93% and hot pepper 54% more grain yield than no treatment. Percentage parasitism (~40%) of aphids was greater on pirimicarb treated plots than on other treatments (<20%). The low percentage on pirimicarb treated plots must be because the aphids are less in number (density-dependent scenario) and parasitism is calculated on the basis of the total number of aphids counted. Parasitism was essentially a late season occurrence. Despite the high prevalence of parasitism, parasitoids could not spare the crop from destruction because they just acted late. However, their presence is still valued because otherwise these crops would have been abandoned altogether. More interestingly, predatory coccinellids were more on hot pepper and garlic treated plots than on pirimicarb treated plots (Wale, 2004). Grain yield was positively correlated with the level of aphid parasitism, coccinelid number and number of pods per plant and strongly negatively with aphid density. Because the objective of the experiment was finding good botanical against pea aphids, hot pepper was found better candidate.

Summary and Conclusion

Biology and ecology studies show that lentil is the most suitable of the legumes for the development of the pea aphid. Thus lentils may not be good choice of crop in places where pea aphids is a problem. It is, however, suitable for use in mass rearing of aphids for resistant variety selection or for natural enemy mass production. A prolonged developmental period and short reproductive period of the aphid may be used as criteria for resistant crop variety selection.

Pea aphids infested the cultivated forage crop, vetch, the wild legume, clover, and the perennial tree, pigeon pea, but not the cultivated lupine and alfalfa. Causes may include differences in aphid biotype that have developed specifically to each host plant, differences in secondary metabolites or alkaloids that deter pests or the level of nitrogen content of the plants. Given the limited research attention given to this group of pests in Ethiopia, the studies so far conducted prompt us to ask more questions than give definitive conclusion of issues. All of these issues are just speculations which need to be verified by further research. Biotypes, metabolites and nitrogen content are subject for study, which students or researchers can pick.

The population dynamics studies at the study sites indicate that pea aphid numbers rise in August at the cooler area, an intermediate altitude in the Ethiopian context, and mostly in September at the warmer area. For optimal yields planting peas from mid- to late June and at the first week of June at the warmer place is suggested.

The number of nymphs produced and the survival rate of adult aphids steadily declined as aphid density per plant increased. Survival and reproduction was the lowest on faba bean across all levels of aphid density per plant.

Compared to the untreated control, primicarb and hot pepper treated grass pea generally had less aphid abundance and had more grain yield. Further trials on the rate and frequency of application are needed to determine the cost-effectiveness of treatments alone or in combination with other products such as soaps or kerosene. Garlic and hot pepper are well known cash crops grown and it may be unlikely that growers will use these crops for the control of pea aphids on such marginal crops as grass pea. In the study area, farmers must grow grass pea in such pea aphid hotspot area every other year for the sole purpose of crop rotation, otherwise, as farmers know from experience, their major cereal crops such as wheat and the local staple cereal grain crop, i.e., teff (*Eragrostis tef* Zucc. Trotter), will fail. Even if there is no grass pea yield at all due to pea aphids, farmers continue growing it for soil amelioration. Many farmers also spray insecticides to control pea aphids to be able to get some yield, though it proved too difficult to stop the aphids even with frequent sprays.

Because in the host preference study pea aphids occurred more on grass pea and field pea than on faba bean and lentils, these aphids may be reared on the better performing plant species when the aphids are needed for some studies while it would be advisable to avoid cultivating them in areas where pea aphids are endemic.

References

Abate, T. 1991. Entomophagous arthropods of Ethiopia: A catalog. Technical Manual No. 4. Institute of Agricultural Research, Addis Ababa, Ethiopia. 50 PP.

Abebe, T.; Birhane, T.; Nega, Y. and Workineh, A. 2014. The prevalence and importance of faba bean diseases with special consideration to the newly emerging "Faba Bean Gall" in Tigray, Ethiopia. *Discourse Journal of Agriculture and Food Sciences* 2(2): 33-38.

Abate, T.; Gebremedhin, T. and Ali, K. 1982. Arthropod pests of grain legumes in Ethiopia: Their importance and distribution. Institute of Agricultural Research, Addis Ababa, Ethiopia, 56 pp.

ARC (Adet Research Center). 2011. Research Achievements: A quarter century-long effort to lift the living standards of farmers. Adet Research Center, Bahir Dar, Ethiopia. Pp 117.

Ali, K. and Gebremedhin, T. 1990. Pea aphid: An important pest of field pea. *IAR Newsletter of Agricultural Research* 5(1): 1-2.

Andarge, A. and Birhan, A. 1998. Research on insect pests and diseases in North Shewa. Agricultural Research and technology Transfer Attempts and Achievements in Northern Ethiopia. Proceedings of the Fourth Technology Generation, Transfer and Gap Analysis Workshop, 18-21 March 1997, Bahir Dar, Ethiopia, pp. 140-155, (Seboka, B. and Deresa, A., eds.). Ethiopian Agricultural research Organization (EARO), Addis Ababa, Ethiopia.

Archibald, R. D. 1979. Some observationS on the hosts and distribution of pea aphid, *Acyrthosiphon pisum* (Homoptera: Aphididae) during its establishment in New Zealand. *New Zealand Entomologist* 7(1): 86.

Autrique, A.; Stary, P. and Ntahimpera, L. 1989. Biological control of pest aphids by hymenopterous parasitoids in Burundi. *FAO Plant protection Bulletin* 37(2): 71-76.

Bournoville, R.; Smon, J. C.; Badenhausser, I.; Girousse, C.; Guilloux, T. and Andres, S. 2000. Clones of pea aphid *Acyrthosiphon pisum* (Hemiptera: Aphididae) distinguished using genetic markers differ in their damaging effect on resistant alfalfa cultivars. *Bulletin of Entomological Research* 200(90): 33-39.

Cardona, C.; Fam, E. Z.; Bishara, S. I. and Bushara, A. G. 1984. Field guide to major insect pests of faba bean in the Nile Valley. Information Bulletin No. 2. International Center for Agricultural Research in the Dry Areas (ICARDA). ICARDA, Aleppo, Syria.

Crowe, T. J. and Ali, K. 1983. A checklist of aphids (Homoptera: Aphididae) recorded in Ethiopia. IAR Entomological Bulletin No.3, second revised edition. Institute of Agricultural Research, Addis Ababa, Ethiopia, 9 pp.

Ellsbury, M. M. and Nielsen, M. W. 1981. Comparative host plant range studies of blue alfalfa aphid, *Acyrthosiphonkondoi* Shinji and the pea aphid, *Acyrthosiphonpisum* (Harris) (Homoptera: Aphididae). Technical Bulletin, Science and Education Administration, United States Department of Agriculture, No. 1639, 14 pp.

Davidson, R. H. and Lyon, W. F. 1987. *Insect pests of farm, garden and orchard*. John Wiley and Sons, New York.

Dent, D. 2000. *Insect pest management*, 2nd ed., CABI Publishing, UK.

Gebremedhin, T. 1990. Loss assessment study for pea aphid (*Acyrthosiphon pisum*) (Harris) infestation of field pea. In Proceedings of the 10th Annual Meeting of the Committee of Ethiopian Entomologists (CEE), 7-9 February 1990, Addis Ababa, Ethiopia. CEE, Addis Ababa. pp 75-83.

Hodek, I. 1967. Bionomics and ecology of predaceous Coccinellidae. *Annual Review of Entomology* 12: 79-104.

Kaakeh, W.; and Ducther, J. D. 1993. Rates of increase and probing behavior of *Acyrthosiphon pisum* (Homoptera: Aphididae) on preferred and non-preferred host cover crops. *Environmental Entomology* 22: 1016-1021.

Morgan, D.; Walters, K. F. A. and Aegerter, J. N. 2001. 2001. Effect of temperature and cultivar on pea aphid, *Acyrthosiphon pisum* (Hemiptera: Aphididae) life history. *Bulletin of Entomological Research* 91(1): 47-52.

Sharma, M. L.; Larrivee, J. M. and Theriault, L. M. 1976. The duration of the larval instarts of the pea aphid, *Acyrthosphonpisum* (Harris) (Aphididae: Homoptera), on peas of the variety Perfection. *Ann. Soc. Entomol.Quebec* 21: 144-146.

Tesfaye, A.; Wale, M. and Azerefegne, F. 2012. Seasonal dynamics of pea aphid, *Acyrthosiphon pisum* (Harris) (Homoptera: Aphididae) and reaction to the performance of grass pea, *Lathyrus sativus* L. in northwestern Ethiopia. *International Journal of Current Research* 4(8): 053-061.

Tesfaye, A.; Wale, M. and Azerefegne, F. 2013. *Acyrthosiphon pisum* (Harris) (Homoptera: Aphididae) feeding preference and performance on cool-season food legumes in northwestern Ethiopia. *International Journal of Pest Management* 59(4): 319-328.

Wale, M. 2002. Population dynamics of the pea aphid, *Acyrthosiphon pisum* (Harris) (Homoptera: Aphididae) on field pea, *Pisum sativum* L. in northwestern Ethiopia. *Insect Science and Its Application* 22(2): 131-137.

Wale, M. 2004. Relative efficacy of some botanicals, detergent and kerosene in controlling the pea aphid, *Acyrthosiphon pisum* (Harris) (Hemiptera: Aphididae) on grass pea, *Lathyrus sativus*. *International Journal of Tropical Insect Science* 24(92): 143-149.

Wale, M; Jembere, B. and Seyoum, E. 2000. Biology of the pea aphid *(Acyrthosiphon pisum)* (Harris) (Homoptera: Aphididae) on cool-season legumes. *Insect Science and Its Application* 20(3): 171-2000.

Wale, M; Jembere, B. and Seyoum, E. 2003a. Occurrence of the pea aphid, *Acyrthosiphon pisum* (Harris) (Homoptera: Aphididae) on wild leguminous plants in West Gojam, Ethiopia. *Sinet: Ethiopian Journal of Science* 26(1): 83-87.

Wale, M; Jembere, B. and Seyoum, E. 2003b. Effect of density on reproduction and survival of pea aphid on cool-season food legumes. *Pest Management Journal of Ethiopia* 7: 63-69.

Wegorek, W. and Krzymanska, J. 1975. Biochemical factors of resistance of Lucerne to pea aphid, *Acyrthosiphon pisum*(Harris). *Prace Naukowe Instytutu Ochrony Roslin* 17(2): 19-27.

INDEX

A

B

C

D

E

F

G

H

I

J

K

L

M

N

O

P

Q

R

S

T

U

V

W

X

Y

Z